THE ESSENTIAL MEDITERRANEAN DIET COOKBOOK

300 No-Fuss Recipes.

Quick & Easy Ideas for eating and living well.
Built healthy habits every day.
30-Day Meal Plan for Weight Loss.

Katy Hamilton

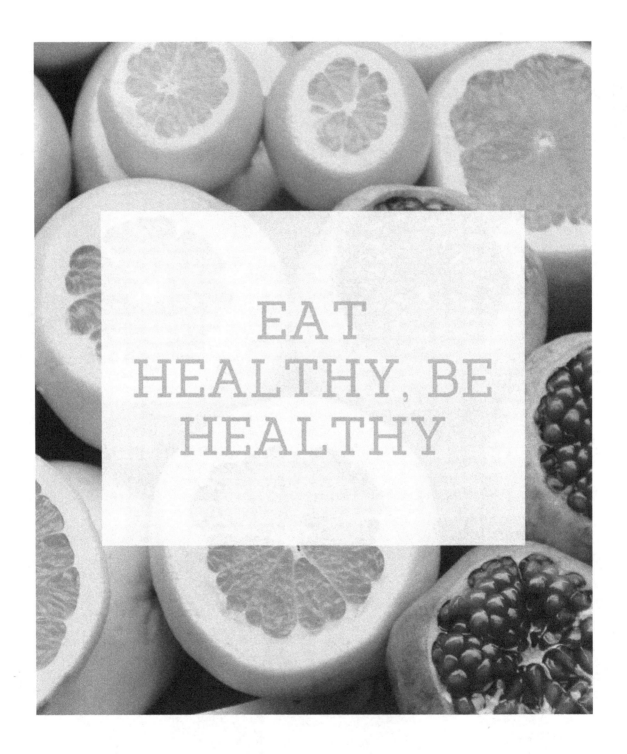

EAT
HEALTHY, BE
HEALTHY

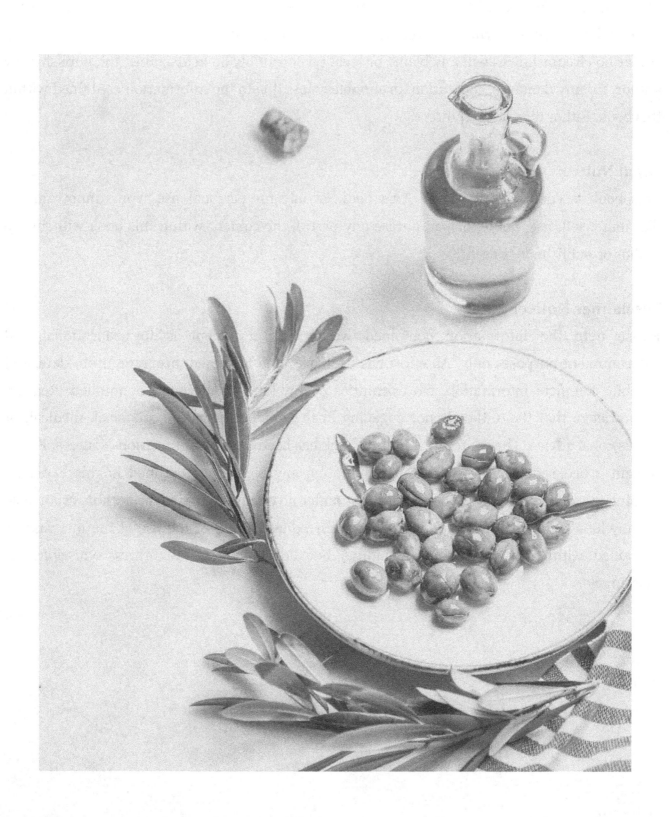

Table of Contents

Table of Contents.................................5

INTRODUCTION 13

UNDERSTANDING THE MEDITERRANEAN DIET 14

The Mediterranean Diet Unchained..............14

THE HISTORY OF MEDITERRANEAN EATING 17

THE SCIENCE BEHIND THE MEDITERRANEAN DIET.......................18

THE PRINCIPLES OF AN AUTHENTIC 19

MEDITERRANEAN DIET............................19

THE MEDITERRANEAN DIET IS A LIFESTYLE....................................19

MORE THAN A DIET.................................19

THE MEDITERRANEAN DIET FOOD PYRAMID 21

WHAT MAKES THE MEDITERRANEAN DIET SO HEALTHY? 22

The Benefit Of The Mediterranean Diet........ 25

HOW TO START THE MEDITERRANEAN DIET 28

HOW TO PLAN YOUR MEDITERRANEAN DIET 29

MEDITERRANEAN SHOPPING GUIDE AND WHERE SHOPPING 32

WHAT FOOD CAN YOU EAT ON MEDITERRANEAN DIET? 33

WHAT FOOD CAN YOU AVOID ON MEDITERRANEAN DIET? 35

What Foods Should You Limit On Mediterranean Diet?......................... 35

THE IMPORTANCE OF OLIVE OIL: BUYING, USING, AND STORING 36

TIPS FOR BUYING...................... 37

STORAGE...............................37

THE IMPORTANCE OF OMEGA-3 (FOODS REACH IN OMEGA-3) 38

What Foods Are Rich In Omega-3.................39

WHAT'S ON YOUR PLATE: HOW TO COMBINE FOODS (CALORIES) –.................41

HOW TO CREATE MEALS AND MENUS 41

TIPS AND TRICKS TO HELP YOU TO FOLLOW 42

THE MEDITERRANEAN DIET.................... 42

HOW TO WEIGHT LOSS 44

30 DAYS MEAL PLAN........................ 45

WEEK 1 45

WEEK 2 47

WEEK 3..50

WEEK 4 52

WEEK 5 54

LET'S START!................................ 55

MEDITERRANEAN RECIPES 55

MEDITERRANEAN BREAKFAST RECIPE .. 55

Creamy Paninis...............................56

Breakfast Couscous..........................56

Potato and Chickpea Hash....................56

Avocado Toast............................... 57

Mediterranean Pancakes 57

Mediterranean Frittata 58

Nutty Banana Oatmeal 59

Mediterranean Veggie Omelet.................. 59

Lemon Scones................................ 59

Breakfast Wrap 60

Garlicky Scrambled Eggs 60

Healthy Breakfast Casserole.................61

Egg and Sausage Breakfast Casserole...........62

Yogurt Pancakes 62

Breakfast Stir Fry.................63

Greek Breakfast Pitas 63

Healthy Breakfast Scramble 64

Greek Parfait.................64

Quiche Wrapped in Prosciutto 64

Morning Couscous.................66

Green Omelet.................66

Healthy Quinoa.................66

MUSHROOM STRAPATSATHA WITH 67

HALLOUMI AND CRISPY BACON.............67

BREAKFAST BAKLAVA FRENCH TOAST ...68

TIGANITES.................68

BEET AND WALNUT MUFFINS 69

FIG JAM 69

HOMEMADE GREEK YOGURT 70

STRAPATSATHA.................70

CHEESE PIES IN YOGURT PASTRY.............71

PAXIMADIA 72

LENTEN PAXIMADIA 72

PAXIMADIA WITH FIGS, STAR ANISE, AND WALNUTS 73

BOUGATSA WITH CUSTARD FILLING 74

FIG, APRICOT, AND ALMOND GRANOLA . 74

GREEK YOGURT SMOOTHIE.................75

GREEK YOGURT WITH HONEY AND GRANOLA 75

GYPSY'S BREAKFAST.................75

BREAKFAST BRUSCHETTA.................76

ROASTED POTATOES WITH VEGETABLES 76

RYE-PUMPERNICKEL STRATA WITH BLEU CHEESE 77

POLENTA 77

FRUIT-STUFFED FRENCH TOAST 77

PASTINA AND EGG 78

MEDITERRANEAN OMELETTE.................78

STOVETOP-POACHED FRESH COD 79

SWEETENED BROWN RICE.................79

CREAMY SWEET RISOTTO.................80

EGGS IN CRUSTY ITALIAN BREAD............80

FRESH TUNA WITH SWEET LEMON LEEK SALSA 80

YOGURT CHEESE AND FRUIT.................81

PANCETTA ON BAGUETTE 81

VEGETABLE PITA WITH FETA CHEESE....82

ISRAELI COUSCOUS WITH DRIED-FRUIT CHUTNEY.................82

ALMOND MASCARPONE DUMPLINGS......83

MULTIGRAIN TOAST WITH GRILLED VEGETABLES.................83

Energizing Breakfast Protein Bars.................83

Fruity Nutty Muesli.................84

Egg Veggie Scramble.................84

MEDITERRANEAN LUNCH RECIPE..........85

Quinoa Salad with Watermelon and Feta......85

Mediterranean Orzo.................86

Meyer Lemon Quinoa Skillet 86

Creamy Corn, Squash and Cilantro 86

Mediterranean Turkey and Rice Skillet........87

Mediterranean Quinoa Stuffed Peppers........87

Japanese Onigiri Rice Triangles Recipe 88

Maple Pumpkin Pie Buckwheat Groats 88

Chicken, Broccoli, and Rice Casserole Recipe 89

Baked Coconut Rice 89

Healthy Butternut Squash Grain Bowl 90

Low Sodium Garlic Parmesan Popcorn 90

Gluten-Free Coconut Granola 91

Simple Black Bean and Barley Vegetarian
Burritos 91

Pecan Brown Butter Oat Triangles Recipe 92

Golden Pilaf 92

Wild Rice Pilaf 93

Moroccan Couscous 93

Couscous with Tomatoes and Cucumbers 94

Charcuterie Bistro Lunch Box 94

Mediterranean Chicken Quinoa Bowl 94

Mediterranean Lettuce Wraps 95

Salmon Pita Sandwich 95

Hummus & Greek Salad 96

Mediterranean Wrap 96

Mediterranean Bento Lunch 97

Greek Chicken & Cucumber Pita Sandwiches
with Yogurt Sauce 97

Slow-Cooker Mediterranean Chicken &
Chickpea Soup 98

Prosciutto, Mozzarella & Melon Plate 98

Mediterranean Pasta Salad 99

Mediterranean Chickpea Quinoa Bowl 99

Mediterranean Lentil & Kale Salad 100

Ravioli & Vegetable Soup 100

Mediterranean Tuna-Spinach Salad 100

Italian Pesto Chicken Salad 101

Edamame & Chicken Greek Salad 101

Tomato, Cucumber & White-Bean Salad with
Basil Vinaigrette 102

Couscous & Chickpea Salad 102

Meal-Prep Roasted Vegetable Bowls with Pesto
.... 102

Beet & Shrimp Winter Salad 103

Creamy Pesto Chicken Salad with Greens ... 103

Tabbouleh, Hummus & Pita Plate 103

Mediterranean Edamame Toss 104

Fig & Goat Cheese Salad 104

White Bean & Veggie Salad 105

Greek-Style Chicken Salad 105

Quinoa Chickpea Salad with Roasted Red
Pepper Hummus Dressing 105

Meal-Prep Falafel Bowls with Tahini Sauce 106

Shrimp, Avocado & Feta Wrap 106

Mediterranean Veggie Wrap with Cilantro
Hummus 106

Vegan Bistro Lunch Box 107

Mediterranean Chicken Salad 108

Edamame Hummus Wrap 108

Tomato Salad with Grilled Halloumi and Herbs
.... 109

Harissa Chickpea Stew with Eggplant and
Millet 109

Grilled Lemon-Herb Chicken and Avocado
Salad 110

5-Minute Heirloom Tomato and Cucumber
Toast 110

Greek Chicken and Rice Skillet 111

Mini Chicken Shawarma 111

Mediterranean feta salad with pomegranate dressing.. 112

Mediterranean scones 113

Spiced baked figs with ginger mascarpone... 113

Crispy squid with caponata 114

Watermelon & feta salad with crispbread 115

Aïoli.. 115

Crunchy baked mussels 116

Easy stuffed peppers.................................... 116

Mediterranean slices.................................... 116

Mediterranean chicken tray bake 117

Mussels with tomatoes & chilli 117

Mediterranean chicken with roasted vegetables 118

Roasted peppers with tomatoes & anchovies118

MEDITERRANEAN LUNCH RECIPE 119

Mediterranean Stuffed Chicken Breasts....... 119

Charred Shrimp & Pesto Buddha Bowls....... 119

Sheet-Pan Salmon with Sweet Potatoes & Broccoli 120

Mediterranean Ravioli with Artichokes & Olives 121

Slow-Cooker Mediterranean Stew................ 121

Greek Cauliflower Rice Bowls with Grilled Chicken 122

Prosciutto Pizza with Corn & Arugula 122

Cheesy Spinach-&-Artichoke Stuffed Spaghetti Squash...123

Vegan Mediterranean Lentil Soup................124

EatingWell's Eggplant Parmesan 124

BBQ Shrimp with Garlicky Kale & Parmesan-Herb Couscous...125

Green Shakshuka with Spinach, Chard & Feta 126

One-Skillet Salmon with Fennel & Sun-Dried Tomato Couscous...................................... 126

Chicken & Spinach Skillet Pasta with Lemon & Parmesan 127

Quinoa, Avocado & Chickpea Salad over Mixed Greens 127

Sheet-Pan Mediterranean Chicken, Brussels Sprouts & Gnocchi 128

Caprese Stuffed Portobello Mushrooms...... 129

Sweet & Spicy Roasted Salmon with Wild Rice Pilaf 129

Zucchini Lasagna Rolls with Smoked Mozzarella... 130

Herby Mediterranean Fish with Wilted....... 130

Chicken with Tomato-Balsamic Pan Sauce .. 131

Roasted Pistachio-Crusted Salmon with Broccoli 132

Crispy Baked Ravioli with Red Pepper & Mushroom Bolognese 132

Pan-Seared Halibut with Creamed Corn & Tomatoes..133

Greek Burgers with Herb-Feta Sauce 134

Greek Roasted Fish with Vegetables........... 134

Easy Pea & Spinach Carbonara....................135

MEDITERRANEAN SALAD RECIPES........ 136

Grilled Tofu with Mediterranean Salad....... 136

Mediterranean Barley Salad 136

Mediterranean Quinoa Salad....................137

Healthy Greek Salad 137

Almond, Mint and Kashi Salad.................... 138

Chickpea Salad.. 138

Italian Bread Salad...................................... 139

Bulgur Salad.. 140

Greek Salad 140

Potato Salad 140

Mediterranean Green Salad......................... 141

Chickpea Salad with Yogurt Dressing 142

Warm Lentil Salad.....................................142

TUNA SALAD WITH TOASTED PINE NUTS
....142

WATERMELON AND FETA SALAD...........143

BULGUR SALAD WITH NUTS, HONEY,
CHEESE, AND POMEGRANATE................143

CREAMY COLESLAW 144

ARUGULA, PEAR, AND GOAT CHEESE
SALAD 144

GREEK VILLAGE SALAD 144

STRAWBERRY AND FETA SALAD WITH
BALSAMIC DRESSING................................145

CREAMY CAESAR SALAD 145

POLITIKI CABBAGE SALAD 146

ARUGULA SALAD WITH FIGS AND SHAVED
CHEESE...146

SPINACH SALAD WITH APPLES AND MINT
....147

POTATO SALAD...148

WARM MUSHROOM SALAD 148

SUN-DRIED TOMATO VINAIGRETTE.......149

CREAMY FETA DRESSING 149

KALAMATA OLIVE DRESSING 149

CUCUMBER AND DILL DRESSING 150

GRILLED EGGPLANT SALAD.....................150

LAHANOSALATA (CABBAGE SALAD) 151

TARAMOSALATA/TARAMA (FISH ROE
SALAD).. 151

GRILLED HALLOUMI SALAD 152

GRILLED BANANA PEPPER SALAD 152

DANDELION GREENS 153

SLICED TOMATO SALAD WITH FETA AND
BALSAMIC VINAIGRETTE..........................153

MEDITERRANEAN POULTRY RECIPES ...153

Chicken Bruschetta 153

Coconut Chicken 154

Turkey Burgers 154

Chicken with Greek Salad 154

Braised Chicken with Olives 155

Braised Chicken with Mushrooms and Olives
....156

Chicken with Olives, Mustard Greens, and
Lemon 156

Delicious Mediterranean Chicken 157

Warm Chicken Avocado Salad......................157

Chicken Stew.. 158

Chicken with Roasted Vegetables.................159

Grilled Chicken with Olive Relish................159

Grilled Turkey with Salsa........................... 160

Curried Chicken with Olives, Apricots and
Cauliflower... 160

Chicken Salad with Pine Nuts, Raisins and
Fennel 161

Slow Cooker Rosemary Chicken 162

CHICKEN SOUVLAKI 162

GREEK-STYLE ROASTED CHICKEN WITH
POTATOES 163

ROAST CHICKEN WITH OKRA 163

CHICKEN CACCIATORE 164

CHICKEN GIOULBASI............................... 165

GRAPE-LEAF CHICKEN STUFFED WITH
FETA 165

GRILLED WHOLE CHICKEN UNDER A
BRICK 166

SKILLET CHICKEN PARMESAN 166

CHIANTI CHICKEN 167

CHICKEN BREASTS WITH SPINACH AND FETA 168

CHICKEN TAGINE WITH PRESERVED LEMONS AND OLIVES 169

POMEGRANATE-GLAZED CHICKEN 170

CHICKEN MASKOULI 170

PESTO-BAKED CHICKEN WITH CHEESE 171

ROSEMARY CHICKEN THIGHS AND LEGS WITH POTATOES 171

ROAST TURKEY 172

TURKEY BREAST PICCATA 172

BACON-WRAPPED QUAIL 173

ROASTED CORNISH HENS STUFFED WITH GOAT CHEESE AND FIGS 173

ROAST LEMON CHICKEN 174

CHICKEN WITH YOGURT 175

CHICKEN WITH EGG NOODLES AND WALNUTS 175

STUFFED GRILLED CHICKEN BREASTS..176

CHICKEN LIVERS IN RED WINE..............176

CHICKEN GALANTINE 177

SPICY TURKEY BREAST WITH FRUIT CHUTNEY 177

GRILLED DUCK BREAST WITH FRUIT SALSA 178

QUAIL WITH PLUM SAUCE 178

SLOW-COOKED DUCK..............................178

GOOSE BRAISED WITH CITRUS 179

SAGE-RICOTTA CHICKEN BREASTS 179

TURKEY TETRAZZINI...............................180

Chicken and Penne 180

MEDITERRANEAN SEAFOOD RECIPES ...181

Salmon and Vegetable Kedgeree 181

Grilled Sardines with Wilted Arugula..........181

Curry Salmon with Napa Slaw 182

Shrimp and Pasta..182

Roasted Fish..183

Baked Fish...183

Spanish Cod 184

Greek Salmon Burgers 184

Grilled Tuna 185

Easy Fish Dish...185

Salmon Bean Stir-Fry 185

Mediterranean Flounder..............................186

Fish with Olives, Tomatoes, and Capers......186

Mediterranean Cod 187

BIANKO FROM CORFU 187

GRILLED SALMON WITH LEMON AND LIME 188

SEA BASS BAKED WITH COARSE SEA SALT 189

BEER-BATTER FISH 189

GRILLED SARDINES................................190

GRILLED WHOLE FISH 190

OLIVE OIL–POACHED COD 191

PLAKI-STYLE BAKED FISH 191

PISTACHIO-CRUSTED HALIBUT.............192

ROASTED SEA BASS WITH POTATOES AND FENNEL.. 192

RED MULLET SAVORO STYLE.................193

SPINACH-STUFFED SOLE 193

GRILLED OCTOPUS 194

SCALLOPS SAGANAKI 195

GRILLED GROUPER STEAKS.................... 195

GRILLED CALAMARI 196

GRILLED LOBSTER.................................... 196

GRILLED JUMBO SHRIMP 196

OCTOPUS STIFADO 197

OYSTERS ON THE HALF SHELL.............. 198

COD WITH RAISINS.................................. 198

AEGEAN BAKED SOLE 198

BAKED SEA BREAM WITH FETA AND
TOMATO 199

BAKED TUNA... 199

BRAISED CUTTLEFISH 200

STOVETOP FISH... 200

GRILLED SEA BASS 201

OCTOPUS IN WINE................................... 201

CIOPPINO 202

STEAMED SNOW CRAB LEGS.................. 202

STEAMED SEAFOOD DINNER.................. 202

GRILLED FISH WITH POLENTA 203

BACCALÁ... 203

FLOUNDER WITH BALSAMIC REDUCTION
.... 204

HALIBUT ROULADE.................................. 204

PARCHMENT SALMON 205

BARBECUED MARINATED TUNA 205

FISH CHILI WITH BEANS 205

SAUTÉED RED SNAPPER.......................... 206

SALMON AND HADDOCK TERRINE........ 206

TILAPIA WITH SMOKED GOUDA............. 207

Grilled Salmon... 207

MEDITERRANEAN MEAT, BEEF AND PORK
RECIPES 208

Liver with Apple and Onion......................... 208

Lamb Chops 209

Sage Seared Calf's Liver 209

Seasoned Lamb Burgers 210

London Broil with Bourbon-Sautéed
Mushrooms 210

Grilled Sage Lamb Kabob 211

Lemony Pork With Lentils............................ 211

Cumin Pork Chops....................................... 212

Healthy Lamb Burgers................................. 213

Herb-Maple Crusted Steak 213

Tenderloin with Blue Cheese Butter........... 214

Green Curry Beef 214

Roasted Pork With Balsamic Sauce.............. 215

Mediterranean Beef Pitas 215

Parmesan Meat Loaf.................................... 216

Mediterranean Flank Steak 216

Mediterranean Lamb Chops 217

LAMB EXOHIKO... 217

LEMON VERBENA RACK OF LAMB.......... 218

TANGY MAPLE-MUSTARD LAMB 219

OSSO BUCO... 219

HÜNKAR BEGENDI WITH LAMB 220

MOUSSAKA 221

SLOW-COOKED PORK CHOPS IN WINE.. 221

PORK CHOPS IN WINE.............................. 222

BREADED PORK CHOPS............................ 222

SMYRNA SOUTZOUKAKIA 223

STUFFED PEPPERS WITH MEAT 223

ROAST PORK BELLY AND POTATOES..... 224

GREEK-STYLE RIBS................................... 225

GRILLED LAMB CHOPS 225

KONTOSOUVLI....................................... 226

PORK SOUVLAKI..................................... 226

SPETSOFAI 227

FASOLAKIA WITH VEAL 227

SLOW-ROASTED LEG OF LAMB............... 228

BRAISED SHORT RIBS KOKKINISTO 228

LAMB ON THE SPIT................................. 229

CABBAGE ROLLS..................................... 230

ZUCCHINI STUFFED WITH MEAT AND
RICE...231

GREEK-STYLE FLANK STEAK 232

CHEESE-STUFFED BIFTEKI 232

MEATBALLS IN EGG-LEMON SAUCE...... 233

AUBERGINE MEAT ROLLS 233

PORK WITH LEEKS AND CELERY............ 234

STIFADO (BRAISED BEEF WITH ONIONS)
.... 235

BRAISED LAMB SHOULDER..................... 235

APRICOT-STUFFED PORK TENDERLOIN 236

STEWED SHORT RIBS OF BEEF............... 236

SICILIAN STUFFED STEAK....................... 236

SAUSAGE PATTIES 237

Healthy Beef and Broccoli 238

MEDITERRANEAN PIZZA RECIPES......... 238

Mediterranean Veggie Pizza 238

Turkish-Style Pizza 239

INTRODUCTION

The term "diet" for most of us spells out deprivation, extreme hunger, and bland and boring foods that we are forced to eat to lose weight. However, with the Mediterranean diet, none of those apply.

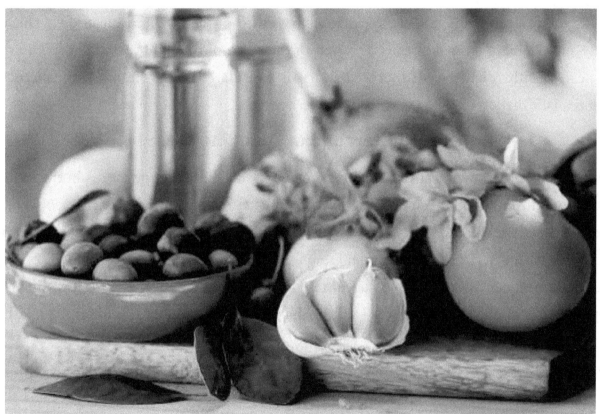

The Mediterranean diet is endowed with an unlimited assortment of fresh, healthy, natural, and wholesome foods from all food groups. Although there is a greater focus on certain ingredients, no natural ingredients are excluded.

Mediterranean diet devotees can enjoy their favorite dishes as they learn to appreciate how nourishing the freshest healthy and natural foods can be.

This diet is primarily based on the eating habits of the original inhabitants of the coasts of Greece, Italy, Spain, Morocco, and France. Their temperate climate and location, seasonal fresh fruit, vegetables, and seafood from these regions' nutritional foundation.

The simplest way to understand the Mediterranean diet is to picture eating as though it's summer every day. It might also give you a déjà vu moment by reminding you of the foods you enjoyed most on a summer vacation or at the beach. In truth, there is never a dull moment with the Mediterranean diet!

All fun aside, the Mediterranean diet will help you find great pleasure in food, knowing that every bite you take will provide your body with the healthiest nutrition.

UNDERSTANDING THE MEDITERRANEAN DIET

Unless you've been living under a rock, you have heard of the Mediterranean diet. This diet has received a lot of press over the last couple of years, all for the right reasons. Also known as the heart-healthy diet, the Mediterranean diet is considered to be the most nutritious and most realistic diet on the planet.

The Mediterranean Diet Unchained

If we take an in-depth look at the Mediterranean diet, it's not a diet per se, as in the sense of being a weight-loss tool—it's more of a lifestyle and a culinary tradition for the people of the Mediterranean region. Its main focus is on whole grains, fresh fruit and vegetables, seafood, nuts, olive oil, and a glass of wine now and then.

The Mediterranean diet is part of a culture that appreciates the freshest ingredients, is prepared in a simple but tasty way, and is shared with friends and family in a laid-back environment.

Most of us understand the importance of eating a clean and well-balanced diet for improved health and better quality of life, but very few of us put this into practice. With most of us spending a greater percentage of our days at work, we tend to opt for fast and easy options for the food we eat. In fact, in many cases, fast food, frozen dinners from food stores, and processed foods are our first options.

Over the years, people worldwide have stopped eating seasonal foods because we can now access all kinds of food all year round. What's more, cooking meals from scratch seems an unnecessary hassle, considering our overburdened schedules and the time it takes to make a good meal.

As a result, we eat foods made in a plant instead of food that grows like a plant. Our diets are characterized by over-processed foods, unhealthy fats, truckloads of sugar, and lots and lots of artificial ingredients, the names of which most of us can't even pronounce.

Perhaps one of the greatest attributes of the Mediterranean diet is that it is very simple and straightforward. You don't need to be a celebrity chef to make the tastiest meals, as you will find in our recipes section. Eat less red meat and instead eat more fish—especially fatty fish rich in omega-3 fatty acids—cook with extra virgin olive oil, and eat fresh fruit, vegetables, whole grains, and nuts several times a day.

Unlike many popular diets, many of which are fads, the Mediterranean diet encourages healthy fats from olive oil, fish, avocado, nuts, and seeds.

For a quick round-up of the Mediterranean diet:

❖ Eat A Plant-Centered Diet

You should build your meals around fresh and organic fruits, vegetables, legumes, nuts, and beans. These whole foods will provide your body with top-grade nutrition in the form of fiber-rich complex carbs that are slow-digesting, as well as antioxidants, vitamins, and phytochemicals.

Additionally, these foods will keep you full longer due to their high fiber content and thus will help keep you from snacking on unhealthy food while providing you with disease-fighting nutrition at the same time.

❖ Only Eat Whole Grains.

Avoid refined grain products such as white rice and bleached white flour, stripped of most of their healthful nutrients. Instead, go for wholegrain products such as oats, brown rice, whole wheat, bulgur, farro, barley, quinoa, millet corn, and so on. Whole grains are higher in fiber, minerals, and vitamins.

❖ Eat Fish Or Shellfish At Least Two Times A Week.

Fish and shellfish are very low in saturated fat, and they provide your body with essential omega-3 fatty acids. In the Mediterranean diet, popular fish and shellfish include clams, anchovies, salmon, mussels, bream, octopus, sardines, shrimp, herring, crab, squid, tuna, and sea bass.

However, make sure you only source wild-caught fish to avoid the mercury contamination common in farmed fish.

❖ Eat Small Portions Of Red Meat Every Once In A While

Red meat is very high in saturated fat. While we include it in the Mediterranean diet for its health benefits, you should eat it in moderation.

Eat as little dairy as possible and limit it to cheese and yogurt.

When consumed in moderation, cheese and natural yogurt are a very healthy part of the Mediterranean diet. These ensure you get enough calcium to promote healthy bones. Yogurt also supplies your body with probiotics that aid digestion by populating your gut with healthy bacteria.

❖ Get Your Healthy Fats From Olives, Avocado, Fatty Fish, Nuts, Seeds, And Olive Oil.

Olives and olive oil, in general, are rich in monounsaturated fats and antioxidants that promote heart health. Eat olives as a snack or add them to stews, salads, or pasta dishes. Avocado is also rich in unsaturated fats. You can eat it as-is or use it in a smoothie or salad.

Nuts and seeds such as almonds, walnuts, hazelnuts, cashews, pine nuts, sesame seeds, and pumpkin seeds are good sources of healthy fats.

Avoid saturated fats found in cream, butter, lard, and red meat, as well as trans fats that are found in margarine or hydrogenated oils.

❖ Drink An Occasional Glass Of Red Wine

When taken in moderation, red wine may improve your heart's health by boosting good cholesterol levels (HDL), which can be attributed to special antioxidants found in red wine.

It's all about moderation.

Though no food is strictly off-limits, it's important to watch what you are eating, as well as your portion sizes, especially when eating foods containing high levels of saturated fat and high-calorie foods. Try as much as possible to eat natural and wholesome food for improved health.

❖ Take Time To Be Physically Active And Enjoy Life.

The Mediterranean lifestyle is more relaxed compared to the typical western lifestyle. People in the Mediterranean region take their time to enjoy meals with friends and family. Most walk or ride a bike to work instead of driving, and they take more vacations, thereby reducing stress.

THE HISTORY OF MEDITERRANEAN EATING

The Mediterranean tradition is characterized by a cuisine rich in aroma, colors, and beautiful memories that support the spirit—and taste—of those in tune with nature.

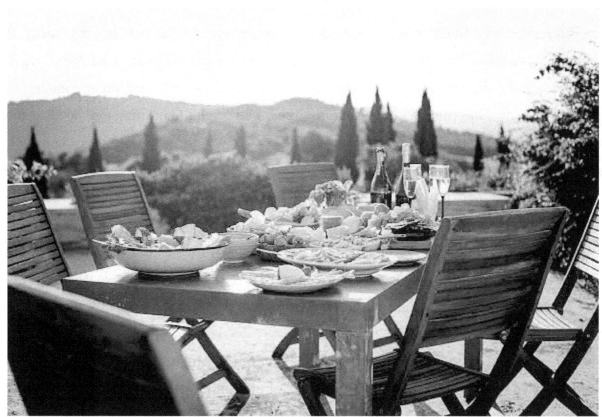

For some time now, everyone has been talking about the Mediterranean diet, but only a handful of people follow it properly. For some, the Mediterranean diet is all about pizza, and for others, it's pasta and meat sauce. This book will look at its beginnings to have a better sense of exactly what the Mediterranean diet entails.

This heart-healthy diet has its origins in the Mediterranean basin, commonly referred to as "The Cradle of Society" because the whole history of the ancient world took place within its geographical borders.

The true origins of the Mediterranean diet are, however, lost in time. We might look back to the eating habits and patterns of the Middle Ages, or even further, to the Roman culture (which modeled the Greek culture) and their identification of red wine, bread, and oil as symbols of their rural culture.

Many people in the Mediterranean region farmed the land and produced fruits and vegetables; they also fished for food. Beef and dairy were not very common in this region, as the climate is not ideal for grazing. Fish, goats, and lamb were the most common protein sources.

THE SCIENCE BEHIND THE MEDITERRANEAN DIET

There is a reason why the Mediterranean diet is often referred to as the "heart-healthy diet." This diet is traditionally high in fresh fruit and vegetables, cereals, and legumes, with moderate fat and dairy consumption and limited meat, saturated fat, and sugar consumption. Most of the fat found in this diet comes from olive oil, avocado, fish, nuts, and seeds. Alcohol is consumed in moderation in the form of red wine.

Scientific research carried out in the 1960s showed that men who adhered to a traditional Mediterranean diet had lower incidences of heart attacks, hence the origin of the "heart-healthy" diet.

Additional investigations have shown that the Mediterranean diet is linked to lower incidences of stroke, cardiovascular disease, type 2 diabetes, and untimely deaths from health issues. Adherence to the principles of the Mediterranean diet has also been shown to improve cognitive ability.

A systemic review carried out to determine the effect of the Mediterranean diet on Dementia showed positive results. The Mediterranean diet offers high antioxidants from the intake of fresh fruit and vegetables and the occasional glass of red wine. These antioxidants may help protect against damage to brain cells associated with Alzheimer's disease and increase the protein levels in your brain that protect your brain cells from damage.

Inflammation is the main culprit behind Alzheimer's disease, and the Mediterranean diet is an effective anti-inflammatory diet. For many of us, the Mediterranean diet is the greatest health insurance policy we can take to guarantee great health.

THE PRINCIPLES OF AN AUTHENTIC

MEDITERRANEAN DIET

1. Cook from scratch, avoid processed foods
2. Eat fresh, seasonal, and where you can, local
3. Get most of your protein from fish and pulses, with eggs and chicken in moderation
4. Get most of your energy from whole grains and potatoes
5. Eat a bit of dairy every day, mostly cheese (sheep and goat is best)
6. Eat red meat occasionally (and mix it in with other ingredients)
7. Enjoy vegetables abundantly
8. Don't be shy with the olive oil
9. Fresh fruit for dessert every day, have cakes, sweets now and again
10. Drink lots of water...and a little wine, if you want to.

THE MEDITERRANEAN DIET IS A LIFESTYLE

MORE THAN A DIET

It might come as a surprise to many that the Mediterranean Diet Pyramid base is not a food group but rather behaviors such as physical activity and social interaction. At its core, the Mediterranean diet is not a diet in the conventional sense of the word. It is a lifestyle that should be enjoyed with both pleasure and health in mind.

❖ **Physical Activity**

The Mediterranean's philosophy of approaching life with an equal measure of pleasure and health leads to a more balanced and happy existence. To most people living in modern urban areas, physical activity means heading off to a gym to work off calories on machines after an entire day's worth of sitting at their desks, in their cars, or on their couches.

To enjoy optimal health and reap the Mediterranean diet rewards, you need to integrate pleasurable forms of activity into their daily lives.

❖ **Camaraderie**

Every country and culture around the Mediterranean has its way of encouraging people to eat together, and family life is valued greatly. Throughout the region's history, eating alone was frowned upon. Only unworthy bachelors or scorned people who didn't have a family would eat by themselves. While attitudes have changed in modern times, most people in the Mediterranean find it unpleasant to eat alone. Fortunately, in many places, work and school schedules revolve around mealtimes. When they do not, families change their schedules to eat together at least for one meal per day.

Residents on the Mediterranean island of Sardinia are ten times more likely to live past 100 than people in the United States. Researchers who studied this remarkable longevity found that daily communal (family style) eat-ing was commonplace and attributed it to residents' overall wellbeing. The researchers concluded that there is something extremely satisfying and comforting about knowing that, no matter how difficult life gets, at lunchtime, you will be surrounded by loved ones. This adds a deep sense of psychological security, which, in turn, has a positive effect on health and happiness.

Throughout the region, food is viewed as a way to express love, thanks, appreciation, and respect. It may be used as a gift, as a way to settle a debt, or as traditional medicine.

I propose simple ways to implement it:

- Vow to live each day with both pleasure and health in mind.
- Find easy, enjoyable ways to get more exercise, such as gardening or walking with a friend.
- Begin incorporating new and varied plant-based foods into your diet.
- Identify simple, make-ahead dishes and snacks to work into your schedule.
- If it is not already a customer, make plans to eat, exercise, and socialize with friends, family, and co-workers as often as possible.
- Treat food, family, and friends as if they are the most important part of your life.

THE MEDITERRANEAN DIET FOOD PYRAMID

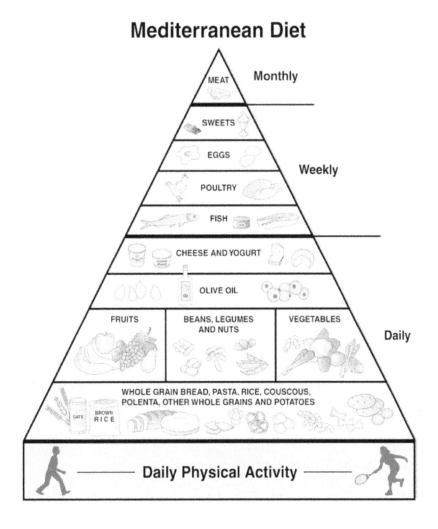

The Mediterranean diet pyramid was developed based on the eating habits of long-living adults in the Mediterranean. It follows a general food pyramid guideline (not specific quantities) and encourages communal eating and an active lifestyle.

"Mediterranean-style diets linked to better brain function in older adults."

- Reduced risk of memory problems and dementia1
- Reduced risk of stroke, diabetes, and other vascular diseases

Base every meal around:

- Vegetables and fruits (the darker in color, the more antioxidants!)
- Legumes/beans, whole grains, nuts (e.g., lentils, walnuts)
- Olive oil as the principal source of fat (swap out margarine and butter!)

Eat at least 2x/week:

- fish, seafood

Eat moderate portions daily to weekly:

- Poultry
- Dairy, cheese, and eggs
- Red wine (typically with meals)

Females: 1 glass/day

Males: 2 glasses/day

Eat less often than other foods:

- Red meat
- Saturated fat
- Sweets

The "Rules."

Fruits, Vegetables, Grains (Mostly Whole), Olive Oil, Beans, Nuts, Legumes & Seeds, Herbs & Spices: These ingredients form the Mediterranean pyramid base, and you should eat some variation of them at every meal.

Fish And Seafood: These are prominent elements of the Mediterranean diet, and you should consume them often—at least two times per week.

Poultry, Eggs, Cheese, And Yogurt: These ingredients are consumed in more moderate amounts in the Mediterranean diet (daily to weekly, depending on the food).

Meats And Sweets: Foods like red meat and sweets are consumed with even less frequency and relatively small quantities in the Mediterranean diet. That's not to say that you shouldn't ever eat red meat or treat yourself to a sweet now and then, but you should do so less often.

WHAT MAKES THE MEDITERRANEAN DIET SO HEALTHY?

1. Eating Slow

As I frequently remind our readers, it isn't just what you eat but also how you eat that counts. People living in Mediterranean climates are renowned for eating patiently, in the company, and taking time to enjoy their food (far from wolfing it down without it touching the sides, which is more of a habit in Western societies!).

Interestingly, research has suggested that even when people who generally live healthier lifestyles have a treat, by being in the habit of eating it more slowly, they may help to protect against some of the adverse effects.

❖ Putting It Into Action

My advice is to give meal times the time and attention they deserve; sit down at a table, with some company if you have family or friends around, and take in the look and scents of your food - getting your mouth watering while making your dinner is also a bonus, another reason to get cooking!

These habits all help to prep your stomach for what's to come. Then, work on chewing slowly and deliberately, preferably reaching 20 chews per mouthful. This will help improve digestion functions, but as you eat slower, you'll feel fuller soon, which will mean you're less likely to overeat - another tick if you're trying to lose a pound or two.

2. Olive Oil

Olive oil is a staple in the Mediterranean diet, and for a good reason. This oil is not only delicious when used in cooking or when drizzling, but it also boasts an array of health benefits. One of the main benefits of olive oil seems to be on the cardiovascular system – pretty major and worth noting as heart disease rates continue to be on the rise (although survival rates have improved).

Research has shown that using olive oil in our diets for just two months could improve blood pressure readings, cholesterol levels, and inflammatory markers, two very impressive indeed!

❖ Putting It Into Action

People often assume that cheaper vegetable oils such as sunflower oil are the best go-to option, but olive oil tends to be a better option all around. Using it in medium temperate cooking is fine (this covers most methods such as sautéing, baking, or roasting), and it's, of course, perfect for drizzling too. One of my top tips is not to shy away from fats. We need a good dose of fats with each meal to help support our metabolism, so don't be afraid to go for that extra drizzle and reap the benefits!

3. Garlic

Garlic is another ingredient that is used generously in a typical Mediterranean diet. It's often used in the bases of sauces, dressings and added to oven-baked dishes to give an extra dose of flavor.

But, other than adding a lovely flavor to dishes, could it also offer some health benefits? Much like olive oil, garlic is also thought to help support our cardiovascular system and lower the risk of high blood pressure, inflammation, and clogged up arteries.3

❖ **Putting It Into Action**

Garlic is much easier to incorporate into your diet if you're cooking from fresh – onion and garlic make an excellent base for almost any dish! Crush or slice your garlic for different strengths and textures, and roasting a garlic bulb in the oven creates a delicious sweetness. Get experimental, and it'll soon become second nature to you to include some garlic in most meals.

4. Vegetables

Although it's hard to pinpoint exactly which element of the Mediterranean diet makes it so especially healthy, I guess it's the combination of different healthy elements that make it so advantageous.

One other element of this diet worth mentioning (plus it's most definitely achievable) is the inclusion of lots of fresh fruit and vegetables. Interestingly, another key point is the types of, and quite simply, the variety included. They tend to include lots more sour and bitter tastes, something we generally lack in Western societies. Bitter-tasting vegetables especially, such as greens, artichoke, or cruciferous veg, will not only supply you with key nutrients, but the taste helps spur your digestion into action, meaning we can digest our food better and make better use of all the nutrients our diet provides – neat!

5. Oily Fish

Rather than being too heavy on meat, Mediterranean diets tend to include more fish, particularly oily varieties, including sardines, mackerel, and fresh tuna.

Oily fish is rich in heart-healthy omega-3. While copious research suggests omega-3 is good for your heart, there's also reason to believe it is also beneficial for our brain function, for managing general inflammation around the body.

Putting It Into Action

As above, incorporating more oily fish into our diets is something you might want to consider working on, especially as you get older. Planning meals in advance each week is an easy way to try to work on incorporating more fish into your regime.

However, if fish isn't your thing, don't worry. There are also plant-based sources of omega-3 available, including walnuts, flaxseeds (don't forget about their oils, too), and avocados.

6. Red Wine

Last, but not least, you may have wondered, because red wine is included generously in a typical Mediterranean diet, if this is something you'd also be able to include guilt-free.

Now, while I don't recommend actively adding alcohol into your diet in a bid to benefit health-wise, there are ways you can approach alcohol to exert the most benefits. After all, red wine contains some antioxidants, including resveratrol, which may benefit the body.

❖ Putting It Into Action

When it comes to alcohol, we need to consider a few key points: how much you are consuming. Secondly, the quality of the alcohol; sipping on some good quality red wine of an evening will be more beneficial than glugging aimlessly on some poor quality vodka.

Finally, how you drink your favorite tipple, drinking it slowly alongside a nutrient-packed dinner, is the way forward, rather than binge drinking on an empty stomach.

The Benefit Of The Mediterranean Diet

❖ Low In Processed Foods And Artificial Sugars

The Mediterranean diet comprises foods that are very close to their naturally occurring state, like olive oil, peas, legumes, fruits, nuts, seeds, vegetables, and unrefined whole grain products. Beyond plant-based foods, another common food is wild-caught fish, with sardines, salmon, and anchovies being the most popular options. Moderate consumption of goat, cow, or sheep cheeses and yogurts is encouraged to receive calcium, healthy fats, and good cholesterol.

While most people in the Mediterranean region are not vegetarian, this diet promotes a very small meat consumption. Choose healthier options that will improve your health and also help you lose weight.

❖ Healthy And Sustainable Weight Loss

If you are looking to shed excess pounds without feeling deprived and keep the weight off for the rest of your life, this is the plan for you. This diet has been undertaken by numerous people with great success, not just in weight loss but also in overall health. It naturally eliminates processed foods and unhealthy fats by focusing on plant-based foods.

Additionally, there's room for interpretation in the Mediterranean diet, whether you prefer to eat a low-protein diet, or a low-carb diet, or a diet that's in between. The Mediterranean diet's main focus is on the consumption of fruits, vegetables, healthy fat, and high-quality protein.

❖ Improves Your Heart Health

Olive oil plays an important role in the Mediterranean diet. Alpha-linoleic acid is a compound found in olive oil and has been shown to reduce the risk of deaths related to cardiac problems by up to 45 percent.

Adherence to the Mediterranean diet, which includes omega-3 and monounsaturated fats, has been shown to reduce mortality linked to heart disease. It lowers high blood pressure and bad cholesterol levels.

Fights Off Cancer

The Mediterranean diet offers a balanced ratio between omega-3 and omega-6 essential fats and a healthy supply of fiber, vitamins, antioxidants, minerals, and polyphenols found in olive oil, fruit, vegetables, and wine.

This antioxidant-rich diet helps fight cancer right, left and center, by protecting your DNA from damage, lowering inflammation, stopping cell mutation, and delaying the growth of tumors.

Olive oil has also been shown to reduce the risk of bowel and colon cancers.

❖ Prevents And Reduces Symptoms Of Diabetes

The Mediterranean diet is the ultimate anti-inflammatory diet, thanks to its emphasis on organic and natural produce. This anti-inflammatory property helps fight chronic diseases associated with chronic inflammation, such as type 2 diabetes.

The Mediterranean diet keeps diabetes at bay by regulating your insulin levels. An excess of insulin, the hormone that controls your blood sugar levels, makes you gain weight and store sugar and other carbohydrates as fat.

When you regulate your blood sugar levels using a healthy diet, your body becomes more efficient at burning fat. This helps you stabilize blood sugar levels and can also help you lose weight.

❖ Improves Mood And Boosts Cognitive Function

This heart-healthy diet is a natural way to preserve your memory, and when followed keenly, it might help prevent and reduce symptoms of Parkinson's disease, Dementia, and Alzheimer's disease. Problems occur when your brain does not receive adequate nutrition to help synthesize dopamine, a hormone responsible for mood regulation, proper body movement, and thought processes.

The healthy nutrition provided by the Mediterranean diet fights off the harmful effects of exposure to toxins and also helps prevent age-related cognitive decline.

❖ Longevity

A fresh, healthy, natural, organic, and wholesome diet means that every system in your body will be operating at optimal capacity, thus giving you newfound energy to carry on with your daily responsibilities. Your skin will improve, your hair will improve. Everything about you will be as good as new!

❖ A Great De-Stressor And Relaxant

The Mediterranean lifestyle is not confined to what you eat; it encourages you to spend quality time with nature and the people you love, such as your family and friends. There's no greater way to have fun with your family than over a delicious and healthy home-cooked meal served outdoors, as you crack jokes and do what you all love to do. Maybe even dance!

Nothing beats a glass of red wine after a meal shared with family.

The Mediterranean diet is a way of life that will improve your overall health, help you lose weight, and find balance in life. It will teach you how to have a deep appreciation for nature and all it offers.

HOW TO START THE MEDITERRANEAN DIET

The Mediterranean diet is an effective way to incorporate healthier foods. Here are the basics:

Fruits And Vegetables: Your meal plates should be covered primarily with a variety of fruits and vegetables. Legumes are also common on the Mediterranean plate, either in salads or soups. This includes kidney beans, garbanzo beans (chickpeas), peas, split peas, and lentils.

Healthy Plant Oils: Mediterranean-style diets include significantly more calories from healthy plant oils, especially extra-virgin olive oil. In Mediterranean cooking, To avoid upset stomachs and bowels, ramp up the amount of oil in your diet gradually.

Use olive oil for salad dressings and for dipping with wholegrain bread. Coat vegetables liberally with olive oil and roast them in the oven. Root vegetables work well, but also eggplant and potatoes.

Eat seeds and nuts, too, as snacks or in salads and grain or pasta dishes and as substitutes for red and processed meat.

Whole Grains: Eat moderate portions of unrefined and wholegrain cereals and bread. (Read the nutrition labels because packaged bread products may contain excessive amounts of sodium.) Other options are whole grain rice or pasta.

Dairy: Eat moderate amounts of yogurt and cheese, mostly as a topping or side dish. Add grated cheese or crumbled feta to leafy salads and cold grain dishes, like bulgur wheat salad (tabbouleh).

Fish: Use fish as the main protein source. Also, enjoy poultry and a moderate number of eggs—up to three or four per week.

Red Meat: A small amount of fresh, unprocessed red meat—one or two portions per week—can fit into a healthy Mediterranean diet. Avoid processed meats containing high sodium or other preservatives, including "low fat" deli meats.

Alcohol: Traditional Mediterranean diets consumed in non-Muslim cultures often include alcohol in moderate amounts, usually with meals. No more than two drinks per day; for women, no more than once per day.

Sweeteners: Avoid sugar-sweetened beverages, baked goods, and rich desserts in large portions that may contain lots of refined carbohydrates and trans fats, which are both unhealthy.

Minimize white bread, white rice, potatoes, and refined carbohydrates such as those found in most breakfast cereals and energy bars. These carbohydrates are quickly digested, producing large rises in blood sugar and insulin that are often indistinguishable from eating simple sugar.

HOW TO PLAN YOUR MEDITERRANEAN DIET

You can do small things that will change your life forever, and they

start with having a clear plan that involves setting goals. However, setting your goals is often the easiest part—it's achieving them that can be a bit of a challenge.

The best way to achieve your goals is to make them into a science: plan, plan and plan. Start with plan A and if it doesn't work, move to plan B and so on, but no matter what, never quit!

❖ **Take It One Step At A Time.**

Take baby steps and focus on one goal at a time. Start with a goal that you are confident you can do every day for the next week: like getting up when your alarm rings without having to use the snooze button or eating fresh vegetables at every meal.

Being successful doesn't only mean achievement; it means you have picked up a new healthy habit. Once you have acquired one, what's to stop you from acquiring more healthy habits?

- Be driven by deadlines, and always write them down.
- Having deadlines will turn you "I wish" into "I did it!"
- Writing down each deadline gives life to your goals and is a very powerful way of committing yourself.
- You now know the principles of the Mediterranean diet. Add a sustainable exercise regimen to these, and you will be on your path to great health.
- Remember to take it one day at a time, and eventually, the Mediterranean diet will be second nature to you.

MONDAY

Breakfast: Bircher muesli

Lunch: Hearty minestrone

Dinner: Grilled lemon and chili chicken with couscous

Pudding: Full of fruit sundaes

Snacks: Greek yogurt, a peach, a medium banana, 30g plain almonds, 40g carrot sticks, and 30g houmous

Milk: 225ml whole milk

TUESDAY

Breakfast: 30g oat flakes with 125g Greek yogurt, 80g raspberries, and 85g banana

Lunch: Salmon, red onion, and sweet pepper wraps

Dinner: Cod Portugaise with boiled new potatoes and a side salad

Pudding: Apple, blackberry, oat, and seed crumble

Snacks: One apple and crunchy peanut butter, two oatcakes with cottage cheese and cucumber, one orange

Milk: 225ml semi-skimmed milk

WEDNESDAY

Breakfast: Bircher muesli

Lunch: Hearty Spanish omelet with salad

Dinner: Galician stew with roasted butternut squash

Pudding: One medium banana

Snacks: Honeydew melon and Greek yogurt, plain almonds, oatcakes, and houmous

Milk: 225ml whole milk

THURSDAY

Breakfast: Two slices of medium granary toast with crunchy peanut butter and a banana

Lunch: Chickpea and tuna salad

Dinner: Greek-style chicken pittas

Pudding: Blackcurrant and raspberry ice cream made with calcium-fortified soya milk

Snacks: Warm exotic fruit salad with Greek yogurt, 50g cottage cheese with 80g cherry tomatoes and 30g pumpkin seeds, one orange

Milk: 225ml semi-skimmed milk

FRIDAY

Breakfast: Very berry porridge

Lunch: Minted aubergine with spinach and pine nuts, paired with grilled chicken breast

Dinner: Crisp salmon salad

Pudding: Apple, blackberry, oat, and seed crumble

Snacks: One peach, Greek yogurt with plain almonds, spicy roasted chickpeas

Milk: 225ml semi-skimmed milk

SATURDAY

Breakfast: Two poached eggs with rye bread and vegetable oil-based spread

Lunch: Roast mackerel with a curried coriander crust with baby new potatoes and broccoli

Dinner: Aubergine and courgette parmesan bake and peas

Pudding: Fruity chocolate traybake

Snacks: 80g raspberries with Greek yogurt, two oatcakes with cottage cheese and cucumber, plain almonds

Milk: 225ml whole milk

SUNDAY

Breakfast: Oat flakes and Greek yogurt with raspberries and banana

Lunch: Hearty minestrone

Dinner: Greek homestyle chicken with Tomato, olive, asparagus, and bean salad

Pudding: Warm exotic fruit salad with Greek yogurt

Snacks: Plain almonds, two satsumas, spicy roasted chickpeas

Milk: 225ml semi-skimmed milk

MEDITERRANEAN SHOPPING GUIDE AND WHERE SHOPPING

You should always choose the least processed foods, with a higher priority being on fresh and organic produce. It's advisable to shop around the grocery store's perimeter: This is usually where whole foods are found.

Here is a simple list you can use the next time you go food shopping:

Fruits: grapes, apples, berries, citrus fruits, avocado, bananas, papaya, pineapple, etc.

Vegetables: broccoli, mushrooms, celery, carrots, kale, onions, leeks, eggplant, etc.

Frozen vegetables: healthy mixed veggie options

Legumes: beans, lentils, peas, etc.

Grains: all whole grains, including wholegrain pasta and wholegrain bread

Nuts: almonds, walnuts, cashews, hazelnuts, pistachios, pine nuts, etc.

Seeds: pumpkin, hemp, sesame, sunflower, etc.

Fish: salmon, tuna, herring, sardines, sea bass, etc.

- Shellfish varieties and shrimp
- Free-range chicken
- Baby potatoes and sweet potatoes
- Cheese
- Natural Greek yogurt
- Olives
- Pastured eggs
- Meat: goat, pork, and pastured beef
- Extra virgin olive oil

As a rule of thumb, eliminate all unhealthy foods not supported by the Mediterranean diet from your kitchen, including candy, refined grain products, sodas, and artificially sweetened beverages, crackers, and other processed foods.

If the only food you have in your home is healthy, that is what you are going to eat. You can't eat what's not there!

WHAT FOOD CAN YOU EAT ON MEDITERRANEAN DIET?

❖ Olive Oil

Per Tablespoon Serving 120 calories, 0 grams (g) protein, 13g fat, 2g saturated fat, 10g monounsaturated fat, 0g carbohydrate, 0g fiber, 0g sugar.

Benefits Replacing foods high in saturated fats (like butter) with plant sources high in monounsaturated fatty acids, like olive oil, may lower the risk of heart disease by 19 percent.

❖ Tomatoes

Per 1 cup, Chopped Serving 32 calories, 1.5g protein, 0g fat, 7g carbohydrates, 2g fiber, 5g sugar

Benefits: They pack lycopene, a powerful antioxidant associated with a reduced risk of some cancers, like prostate and breast. Other components in tomatoes may help reduce the risk of blood clots, thereby protecting against cardiovascular disease.

❖ Salmon

Per 1 Small Fillet 272 calories, 44g protein, 9g fat, 0g carbohydrates, 0g fiber

Benefits: The fatty fish is a major source of omega-3 fatty acids. For good heart health, eating at least two fish meals per week, particularly fatty fish like salmon.

❖ Walnuts

Per 1 oz (14 Halves) Serving 185 calories, 4g protein, 18g fat, 2g saturated fat, 3g monounsaturated fat, 13g polyunsaturated fat, 4g carbohydrate, 2g fiber, 1g sugar.

Benefits: Rich in heart-healthy polyunsaturated fats, these nuts may also favorably impact your gut microbiome (and thus improve digestive health), as well as lower LDL cholesterol.

❖ Chickpeas

Per ½ Cup Serving 160 calories, 10g protein, 2g fat, 26g carbohydrate, 5g fiber

Benefits: The main ingredient in hummus, chickpeas, is a good source of fiber, which carries digestive health and weight loss benefits, and iron, zinc, folate, and magnesium.

❖ Arugula

Per 1 cup: Serving 5 calories, 0.5g protein, 0g fat, 1g carbohydrate, 0g fiber, and 0g sugar.

Benefits: Leafy greens, like arugula, are eaten in abundance under this eating approach. Mediterranean-like diets that include frequent (more than six times a week) consumption of leafy greens has been shown to reduce the risk of Alzheimer's disease.

❖ Pomegranate

Per ½ Cup Serving (Arils) 72 calories, 1.5g protein, 1g fat, 16g carbohydrates, 4g fiber, 12g sugar

Benefits: This fruit, in all its bright red glory, packs powerful polyphenols that act as an antioxidant and anti-inflammatory. It's also been suggested that pomegranates may have anti-cancer properties, too.

❖ Lentils

Per ½ Cup Serving 115 calories, 9g protein, 0g fat, 20g carbohydrate, 8g fiber, 2g sugar.

Benefits: swapping one-half of your serving of a high-glycemic starch (like rice) with lentils helps lower blood glucose by 20 percent.

❖ Farro

Per ¼ Cup (Uncooked) Serving 200 calories, 7g protein. 1.5g fat, 37g carbs, 7g fiber, 0g sugar

Benefits: Whole grains like farro are a staple of this diet. This grain offers a stellar source of satiating fiber and protein. Eating whole grains is associated with a reduced risk of a host of diseases, like stroke, type 2 diabetes, heart disease, and colorectal cancer.

❖ Greek Yogurt

Per 7 oz Container (Low-Fat Plain) 146 calories, 20g protein, 4g fat, 2g saturated fat, 1g monounsaturated fat, 0g polyunsaturated fat, 8g carbs, 0g fiber, 7g sugar.

Benefits: Dairy is eaten in limited amounts, but these foods serve to supply an excellent calcium source. Opting for low- or nonfat versions decreases the amount of saturated fat you're consuming.

WHAT FOOD CAN YOU AVOID ON MEDITERRANEAN DIET?

Let's be real: Many, many foods are processed to some degree. A can of beans has been processed in the sense that the beans have been cooked before being canned. Olive oil has been processed because olives have been turned into oil. But when we talk about limiting processed foods, avoiding things like frozen meals with tons of sodium. You should also limit soda, desserts, and candy. As the adage goes, if the ingredient list includes items that your great-grandparents wouldn't recognize as food, it's probably processed. If you're buying a packaged food that's as close to its whole-food form as possible — such as frozen fruit or veggies with nothing added — you're good to go.

❖ Processed Red Meat

On the Mediterranean diet, you should minimize your intake of red meat, such as steak. What about processed red meat, such as hot dogs and bacon? You should avoid these foods or limit them as much as possible.

❖ Butter

Here's another food that should be limited to the Mediterranean diet. Use olive oil instead, which has many heart-health benefits and contains less saturated fat than butter. Butter has 7 grams of saturated fat per Tablespoon, while olive oil has about 2 grams.

❖ Refined Grains

The Mediterranean diet is centered around whole grains, such as farro, millet, couscous, and brown rice. You'll generally want to limit your intake of refined grains such as white pasta and white bread with this eating style.

❖ Alcohol

When you're following the Mediterranean diet, red wine should be your chosen alcoholic drink. This is because red wine offers health benefits, particularly for the heart. But it's important to limit intake of any type of alcohol to up to one drink per day for women, men older than 65, and up to two drinks daily for men aged 65 and younger. The amount that counts as a drink is 5 ounces of wine, 12 ounces of beer, or 1.5 ounces of 80-proof liquor.

What Foods Should You Limit On Mediterranean Diet?

- Eggs and poultry are occasional foods in moderate portions.
- Cheese and yogurt are traditional Mediterranean foods, also in moderate portions.

THE IMPORTANCE OF OLIVE OIL: BUYING, USING, AND STORING

Like butter and coconut oil, olive oil is a superfood. There's an incredible amount of nutrition packed into every small amount of oil.

And like butter and coconut oil, including it in your regular cooking habits and consuming just a small portion each day will be enough for your body to reap the benefits of the oil over time.

❖ OLEIC ACID

Olive Oil contains 75% oleic acid, a long-chain fatty acid. This omega-9 is thought to aid in the battle against aggressive breast cancer in as little as one Tablespoon each day (although researchers still suggest obtaining oleic acid from other whole foods such as nuts, seeds, beef, eggs, and cheese that can be eaten throughout the day, rather than a single daily dose).

Oleic acid also strengthens the cell membranes in our bodies' blood vessels, allowing them to withstand the pressure put on by the normal blood flow and daily operation of our bodies.

❖ VITAMIN E

Vitamin E is best known for being an antioxidant, as it prevents and repairs the damage done by unstable free-radicals and is required by our bodies to maintain the integrity of the cell membranes of our mucus membranes. It also aids in the skin's healing process and naturally thins the blood, so platelets don't clump abnormally.

❖ POLYPHENOLS

Olive oil contains at least 18 different polyphenols, including some of nature's most powerful antioxidants. Included in the list are some that protect portions of LDL cholesterol from oxidizing in the blood vessels and potentially becoming calcified. Another type slows the growth of unwanted bacteria responsible for digestive tract infections, including ulcers. Some of these polyphenols' long-term benefits include coronary artery disease, degenerative nerve diseases, improved brain function, and diabetes.

❖ OLEOCANTHAL

Oleocanthal is a specific type of polyphenol worth mentioning because of its anti-inflammatory effects (essentially inhibiting two enzymes). Olive oils with a stronger flavor contain more oleocanthal, and in general, 3 1/2 tablespoons of olive oil is equal to a 200mg capsule of ibuprofen. An excellent way to naturally manage the pain and swelling from arthritis.

TIPS FOR BUYING

- Aim to buy extra virgin olive oil labeled "cold pressed." These oils are extracted from olives using only pressure and nothing else.
- Extra virgin olive oil comes from the first press of the fruit and will have the freshest flavor.
- Virgin olive oil comes from the second press. It still tastes fresh and is only extracted using pressure, but it will be slightly more acidic. The difference may or may not be noticeable, so it could be worth experimenting with the two if the price difference is significant.
- A bottle labeled "light" olive oil means that it has been filtered to remove some of the fruit's sediment. It's not a note about calories or fat, only color. Because filtering can remove some of the benefits of olive oil.
- A bottle labeled "pure" is very misleading, and you should not buy these. It's a combination of refined extra virgin, virgin and olive oils that aren't great quality. Sometimes these bottles are just labeled "olive oil" as well.
- Olives are harvested in the fall, and the oil will be on the shelves the following year. Make sure to check the bottle of your olive oil to ensure a harvest date is listed. This way, you know you're not buying old and possibly rancid oil. Plus, you can guesstimate how long you have to use it.

STORAGE

The relatively short shelf life of olive oil (compared to other fats) makes storage very important.

Storing olive oil incorrectly can potentially cause your expensive oil to go rancid much more quickly. Rancid oil not only tastes bad, but it affects the structural integrity of the oil as well.

- The bottle should be glass, dark and opaque (see-through). Avoid clear glass since light can cause the oil to deteriorate faster.
- Seal the bottle when not in use. Like light, air causes the oil to deteriorate as well.
- Store the oil in a cool location, anywhere from 57-70°F. If your kitchen is usually warmer than this, consider a closet, basement, or garage where it's naturally cooler.
- Keeping your oil in a super cute, clear glass bottle with a pouring spout right next to your stove is bad.

- This goes against every rule on the proper storage of olive oil. Don't do this. Dare to be different.

THE IMPORTANCE OF OMEGA-3 (FOODS REACH IN OMEGA-3)

Omega-3 fatty acids are important fats that you must get from your diet.

As your body cannot produce them on its own, you must get them from your diet.

The three most important types are ALA (alpha-linolenic acid), DHA (docosahexaenoic acid), and EPA (eicosapentaenoic acid). ALA is mainly found in plants, while DHA and EPA occur mostly in animal foods and algae.

Common foods high in omega-3 fatty acids include fatty fish, fish oils, flax seeds, chia seeds, flaxseed oil, and walnuts.

Importance Of Omega 3

1. MAY SUPPORT HEART HEALTH

Heart disease is the leading cause of death worldwide.

Cholesterol levels: It can increase levels of "good" HDL cholesterol. However, it does not appear to reduce levels of "bad" LDL cholesterol.

Triglycerides: It can lower triglycerides by about 15–30%

Blood Pressure: Even in small doses, it helps reduce blood pressure in people with elevated levels.

Plaque: It may prevent the plaques that cause your arteries to harden, as well as make arterial plaques more stable and safer in those who already have them

Fatal Arrhythmias: In people who are at risk, it may reduce fatal arrhythmia events. Arrhythmias are abnormal heart rhythms that can cause heart attacks in certain cases.

2. HELP TREAT CERTAIN MENTAL DISORDERS

Your brain comprises nearly 60% fat, and much of this fat is omega-3 fatty acids. Therefore, omega-3s are essential for normal brain function.

Some studies suggest that people with certain mental disorders have lower omega-3 blood levels.

3. MAY AID WEIGHT LOSS

Obesity is defined as having a body mass index (BMI) greater than 30. Globally, about 39% of adults are overweight, while 13% are obese. Obesity can significantly increase your risk of other diseases, including heart disease, type 2 diabetes, and cancer.

omega-3 supplements may improve body composition and risk factors for heart disease in obese people

4. MAY SUPPORT EYE HEALTH

Like your brain, your eyes rely on omega-3 fats. Evidence shows that people who don't get enough omega-3s have a greater risk of eye diseases.

5. MAY REDUCE INFLAMMATION

Inflammation is your immune system's way of fighting infection and treating injuries.

However, chronic inflammation is associated with serious illnesses, such as obesity, diabetes, depression, and heart disease.

Because omega-3 has anti-inflammatory properties, it may help treat conditions involving chronic inflammation.

6. MAY SUPPORT HEALTHY SKIN

Your skin is the largest organ in your body, and it contains a lot of omega-3 fatty acids.

Skin health can decline throughout your life, especially during old age or after too much sun exposure.

7. MAY SUPPORT PREGNANCY AND EARLY LIFE

Omega-3s are essential for early growth and development.

Therefore, mothers need to get enough omega-3s during pregnancy and while breastfeeding.

Fish oil supplements in pregnant and breastfeeding mothers may improve hand-eye coordination in infants. However, it's unclear whether learning or IQ is improved.

Taking Omega-3

supplements during pregnancy and breastfeeding may also improve infant visual development and help reduce the risk of allergies

What Foods Are Rich In Omega-3

- Eat whole, natural, and fresh foods.

- Eat five to ten servings of fruits and vegetables daily and eat more peas, beans, and nuts.

- Increase intake of omega-3 fatty acids by eating more fish, walnuts, flaxseed oil, and green leafy vegetables. An example of meeting the recommended intake of omega-3 fats is to eat two salmon portions a week or 1 gram of omega-3-fatty acid supplement daily.

- Drink water, tea, nonfat dairy, and red wine (two drinks or less daily for men, one drink or less daily for women).

- Eat lean protein such as skinless poultry, fish, and lean cuts of red meat.

- Avoid trans-fats and limit intake of saturated fats. This means avoiding fried foods,

Food/Food Group	Recommended Intake*	Tips
Vegetables	4 or more servings each day (one portion each day should be raw vegetables)	A serving is 1 cup raw or ½ cup cooked vegetables. Eat a variety of colors and textures.
Fruits	3 or more servings each day	Make fruit your dessert
Grains	4 or more servings each day	Choose mostly whole grains. 1 serving = 1 slice bread or ½ cup cooked oatmeal
Fats/Oils	Olive Oil: 4 Tablespoons or more each day	Choose extra virgin olive oil (EVOO) and use in salad dressings and cooking; choose avocado or natural peanut butter instead of butter or margarine
Dried Beans/Nuts/Seeds	Nuts/Seeds: 3 or more servings each week Beans/Legumes: 3 or more servings each week	1 ounce or 1 serving = 23 almonds or 14 walnut halves; 1 serving of beans = ½ cup
Fish and Seafood	2-3 times each week	Choose salmon, sardines, and tuna which are rich in Omega-3 fatty acids
Herbs and Spices	Use daily	Season foods with herbs, garlic, onions and spices instead of salt
Yogurt/Cheese/Egg Poultry	Choose daily to weekly	Choose low-fat yogurt and cheeses; choose skinless chicken or turkey in place of red meat
Alcohol/Wine	Men: 1-2 glasses each day Women: 1 glass each day	Always ask your medical team if alcohol is ok for you to consume.

*Serving sizes should be individualized to meet energy and nutrient needs.
❖ Red meats, processed meats, and sweets should be limited

hard margarine, commercial baked goods, and most packaged and processed snack foods, high-fat dairy and processed meats such as bacon, sausage, and deli meats.

- Limit glycemic foods. Glycemic foods are those made with sugar and white flour, which increase blood sugar levels. Increased blood sugar levels stimulate the pancreas to release insulin. Chronically high insulin levels are believed to cause weight gain as well as atherosclerosis of the arteries.

WHAT'S ON YOUR PLATE: HOW TO COMBINE FOODS (CALORIES)

–

HOW TO CREATE MEALS AND MENUS

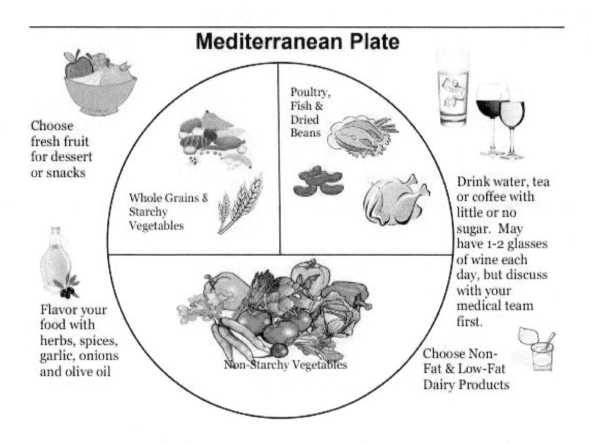

Mediterranean Plate

Choose fresh fruit for dessert or snacks

Flavor your food with herbs, spices, garlic, onions and olive oil

Whole Grains & Starchy Vegetables

Poultry, Fish & Dried Beans

Non-Starchy Vegetables

Drink water, tea or coffee with little or no sugar. May have 1-2 glasses of wine each day, but discuss with your medical team first.

Choose Non-Fat & Low-Fat Dairy Products

TIPS AND TRICKS TO HELP YOU TO FOLLOW

THE MEDITERRANEAN DIET

The Mediterranean diet, which emphasizes fruit and vegetables, grains, nuts, and olive oil is recognized as the gold standard eating pattern promoting good health.

The diet helps guard against heart disease, certain cancers, obesity, diabetes, asthma, Parkinson's, and Alzheimer's disease. And it's been shown to increase life expectancy.

The Mediterranean diet is a diet pattern that's low in saturated fat, high in monounsaturated fat, high in fiber, and packed with protective phytochemicals. The Med diet is primarily plant-based, with fruits, vegetables, whole grains, legumes, and nuts eaten daily.

Dairy products - cheese and yogurt - are also part of the daily diet. Red meat is not. Meat is eaten no more than a few times per month. Poultry and fish are the protein foods of choice and are consumed at least twice per week. The diet also allows up to 7 eggs per week, including those used in cooking and baking.

The principal fat is olive oil; butter and margarine are seldom used. Herbs and spices are used to flavor foods rather than salt.

Scientists speculate the Mediterranean diet's health benefits are due to its strong antioxidant and anti-inflammatory effects.

Use the following eight strategies to help you adopt a Mediterranean-style diet.

❖ Make Fruit And Vegetables Daily Staples

These foods deliver fiber, vitamins, minerals, antioxidants, and phytochemicals and should be eaten at most meals.

Include whole fresh fruit at breakfast, at snacks, and serve fruit salad or berries for dessert. Limit 100% fruit juice to ½ cup per day.

Make sure lunch includes at least one vegetable serving such as a spinach salad, grated raw carrot or beets in a sandwich, red pepper sticks, or vegetable soup. Aim to cover half your plate at dinner with vegetables.

❖ Switch To Whole Grain

Minimally processed grains such as barley, bulgur, couscous, rice, pasta, polenta, farro, millet, and oats are a central part of the Mediterranean diet.

Choose 100% whole grain bread and cereals. Eat brown rice and wholegrain pasta more often than white.

❖ Enjoy Low-Fat Dairy

These foods supply protein, calcium, and B vitamins. Choose low fat (1% milkfat) or nonfat yogurt, or Greek yogurt. Eat cheese in small portions; look for part-skim versions (less than 20% milkfat).

❖ Eat Fish Twice Weekly

To get heart-healthy omega-3 fatty acids, aim to eat oily fish twice per week. Good choices include salmon, sardines, herring, and trout. Enjoy (unbreaded) fish baked, grilled, or steamed.

❖ Scale Back Red Meat

The Mediterranean diet includes lean red meat no more than three times per month (maximum of 12 to 16 ounces per month). Instead of having a large steak, have smaller portions of meat in a stir-fry, vegetable stew, or pasta dish. As the main course, limit your portion to 3 ounces - this fills only one-quarter of your dinner plate.

❖ Add Vegetarian Meals

To increase your intake of vegetarian protein, eat a legume-based meal at least twice per week.

Try a hearty lentil soup, vegetarian chili, black bean tacos, or pasta with white kidney beans.

❖ Choose Healthy Fats

The majority of fats in the diet should be monounsaturated. Use olive oil in cooking and baking. (Extra virgin olive oil is not suitable for high heat frying.) Include one small handful of nuts such as almonds, pecans, and cashews in your daily diet. Instead of butter or margarine, add sliced avocado to sandwiches.

❖ Drink In Moderation

The Med diet typically includes a moderate amount of wine which is consumed with meals. This means no more than 5 ounces per day for women and 10 ounces for men.

 Wine is optional; alcohol, even in moderation, is not healthy for everyone.

HOW TO WEIGHT LOSS

The Mediterranean diet, which focuses on plant foods, like vegetables and fruits, whole grains, pulses, nuts, seeds, and items like pasta and extra virgin olive oil, is consistently ranked by experts as the healthiest way to eat. Although it isn't intended to be a weight-loss plan, following the Mediterranean diet may be a realistic and sustainable way to lose weight and maintain your results. Here's why you may want to consider the Mediterranean diet for weight loss

How To Follow The Mediterranean Diet For Weight Loss

The only thing you need to do to get started is to get organized and plan your menu. Here are some pointers:

Choose Two Breakfasts. Most people are used to eating breakfasts on repeat, so the only change here might be the type of breakfast you're eating. Easy Mediterranean diet options include oatmeal, Greek yogurt, and eggs. Be sure you're eating fruits, veggies, or a mix of both at breakfast.

Decide On Two To Three Easy Lunches And Dinners. When you limit your options, you also narrow the number of ingredients you need to buy and the number of meals you need to cook. Using this strategy, you'll make efficient use of your kitchen time, enjoy some variety, and get some nights off by incorporating leftovers. Each week, you can select different things to make, so your menu continues to feel exciting and enjoyable.

Keep Foods Simple. If you're a less experienced cook, choose low-fuss ingredients, like salad greens, frozen veggies, eggs, canned tuna, and canned or boxed pulses (such as chickpeas and steamed lentils). Simple wholegrain options include quinoa, brown rice, and oats.

Prepare Your Snacks. Whether you're prepping them in advance or making them on demand, replace packaged snacks with whole-food snacks. Fast options include a piece of fruit with nuts or sliced veggies with hummus or olive tapenade.

Focus On The Enjoyment Of Food. No food is forbidden on a Mediterranean diet. Instead, food is appreciated, and meals are designed to be enjoyed. This factor is often missing on weight-loss plans but is an important part of building a healthy relationship with food and sustainable eating habits.

30 DAYS MEAL PLAN

WEEK 1

Day 1

Breakfast: 1 serving Pineapple Green Smoothie (297 calories)

A.M. Snack: 3/4 cup raspberries (48 calories)

Lunch: 1 serving Mediterranean Tuna-Spinach Salad (375 calories)

P.M. Snack: 3/4 cup blackberries (46 calories)

Dinner: 1 serving Dijon Salmon with Green Bean Pilaf (442 calories)

Daily Totals: 1,209 calories, 73 g protein, 123 g carbohydrates, 31 g fiber, 53 g fat, 1,412 mg sodium.

Day 2

Breakfast: 1 serving Muffin-Tin Quiches with Smoked Cheddar & Potato (238 calories)

A.M. Snack: 3/4 cup raspberries (48 calories)

Lunch: 1 serving Instant Pot White Chicken Chili Freezer Pack with a side of 2 celery stalks and 3 Tbsp. hummus (346 calories)

P.M. Snack: 2 plums (61 calories)

Dinner: 1 serving Chicken & Vegetable Penne with Parsley-Walnut Pesto (514 calories)

Daily Totals: 1,206 calories, 75 g protein, 126 g carbohydrates, 32 g fiber, 50 g fat, 1,996 mg sodium.

Day 3

Breakfast: 1 serving Muffin-Tin Quiches with Smoked Cheddar & Potato (238 calories)

A.M. Snack: 1 peach (68 calories)

Lunch: 1 serving Instant Pot White Chicken Chili Freezer Pack with a side of 2 celery stalks and 3 Tbsp. hummus (346 calories)

P.M. Snack: 3/4 cup blackberries and 6 walnut halves (125 calories)

Dinner: 1 serving Greek Turkey Burgers with Spinach, Feta & Tzatziki with a side of 2 cups mixed greens topped with 1 Tbsp. Basil Vinaigrette (442 calories)

Daily Totals: 1,219 calories, 78 g protein, 118 g carbohydrates, 32 g fiber, 54 g fat, 2,205 mg sodium.

Day 4

Breakfast: 1 serving Muffin-Tin Quiches with Smoked Cheddar & Potato (238 calories)

A.M. Snack: 2 plums (61 calories)

Lunch: 1 serving Instant Pot White Chicken Chili Freezer Pack with a side of 2 celery stalks and 3 Tbsp. hummus (346 calories)

P.M. Snack: 1 large peach (68 calories)

Dinner: 1 serving Meal-Prep Falafel Bowls with Tahini Sauce (500 calories)

Daily Totals: 1,213 calories, 59 g protein, 143 g carbohydrates, 31 g fiber, 51 g fat, 2,134 mg sodium.

Day 5

Breakfast: 1 serving Pineapple Green Smoothie (297 calories)

A.M. Snack: 2 plums (61 calories)

Lunch: 1 serving Instant Pot White Chicken Chili Freezer Pack with a side of 2 celery stalks and 3 Tbsp. hummus (346 calories)

P.M. Snack: 3/4 cup blueberries (63 calories)

Dinner: 1 serving Vegetarian Spaghetti Squash Lasagna with a side of 2 cups mixed greens topped with 1 Tbsp. Basil Vinaigrette (416 calories)

Meal-Prep Tip: Prepare 1 serving of Creamy Blueberry-Pecan Overnight Oatmeal to have for breakfast tomorrow

Daily Totals: 1,183 calories, 62 g protein, 170 g carbohydrates, 38 g fiber, 37 g fat, 1,901 mg sodium.

Day 6

Breakfast: 1 serving Creamy Blueberry-Pecan Overnight Oatmeal (291 calories)

A.M. Snack: 3/4 cup raspberries (48 calories)

Lunch: 1 serving Mediterranean Tuna-Spinach Salad (375 calories)

P.M. Snack: 3/4 cup blackberries (46 calories)

Dinner: 1 serving Hasselback Caprese Chicken with 1 1/2 cups Roasted Fresh Green Beans (443 calories)

Daily Totals: 1,203 calories, 77 g protein, 116 g carbohydrates, 34 g fiber, 55 g fat, 1,458 mg sodium.

Day 7

Breakfast: 1 serving Pineapple Green Smoothie (297 calories)

A.M. Snack: 2 plums (61 calories)

Lunch: 1 serving Mediterranean Tuna-Spinach Salad (375 calories)

P.M. Snack: 1 cup sliced cucumbers with squeeze of lemon juice and salt & pepper to taste (16 calories)

Dinner: 1 serving Stuffed Sweet Potato with Hummus Dressing (472 calories)

Daily Totals: 1,221 calories, 61 g protein, 184 g carbohydrates, 40 g fiber, 34 g fat, 1,587 mg sodium.

WEEK 2

Day 8

Breakfast: 1 serving Muffin-Tin Quiches with Smoked Cheddar & Potato (238 calories)

A.M. Snack: 1 cup sliced cucumber with a squeeze of lemon juice and salt & pepper to taste (16 calories)

Lunch: 1 serving Stuffed Sweet Potato with Hummus Dressing (472 calories)

P.M. Snack: 1 plum (30 calories)

Dinner: 1 serving Roasted Root Veggies & Greens over Spiced Lentils (453 calories)

Meal-Prep Tip: Prepare 1 serving of Creamy Blueberry-Pecan Overnight Oatmeal to have for breakfast tomorrow

Daily Totals: 1,209 calories, 54 g protein, 157 g carbohydrates, 39 g fiber, 45 g fat, 1,622 mg sodium.

DAY 9

Breakfast: 1 serving Creamy Blueberry-Pecan Overnight Oatmeal (291 calories)

A.M. Snack: 1/2 cup raspberries (32 calories)

Lunch: 1 serving Roasted Veggie & Quinoa Salad (351 calories)

P.M. Snack: 1/2 cup sliced cucumber with a pinch of salt & pepper (8 calories)

Dinner: 1 serving One-Skillet Salmon with Fennel & Sun-Dried Tomato Couscous (543 calories)

Daily Totals: 1,225 calories, 59 g protein, 143 g carbohydrates, 27 g fiber, 51 g fat, 1,130 mg sodium.

Day 10

Breakfast: 1 serving Everything Bagel Avocado Toast with a side of 1 hard-boiled egg (250 calories)

A.M. Snack: 1 cup raspberries (64 calories)

Lunch: 1 serving Roasted Veggie & Quinoa Salad (351 calories)

P.M. Snack: 5 oz. nonfat plain Greek yogurt (84 calories)

Dinner: 1 serving Mediterranean Chickpea Quinoa Bowl (479 calories)

Meal-Prep Tip: Thaw the Slow-Cooker Pasta e Fagioli Soup Freezer Pack in the fridge overnight. Place in the slow cooker tomorrow morning so it's ready in time for dinner.

Daily Totals: 1,227 calories, 50 g protein, 127 g carbohydrates, 30 g fiber, 59 g fat, 1,390 mg sodium.

Day 11

Breakfast: 1 serving Muesli with Raspberries (287 calories)

A.M. Snack: 1 large peach (68 calories)

Lunch: 1 serving Roasted Veggie & Quinoa Salad (351 calories)

P.M. Snack: 1 plum (30 calories)

Dinner: 1 serving Slow-Cooker Pasta e Fagioli Soup Freezer Pack (457 calories)

Daily Totals: 1,193 calories, 59 g protein, 158 g carbohydrates, 33 g fiber, 44 g fat, 1,116 mg sodium.

Day 12

Breakfast: 1 serving Everything Bagel Avocado Toast with a side of 1 hard-boiled egg (250 calories)

A.M. Snack: 1 cup blackberries (62 calories)

Lunch: 1 serving Roasted Veggie & Quinoa Salad (351 calories)

P.M. Snack: 1 cup nonfat plain Greek yogurt with 1 Tbsp. chopped walnuts (181 calories)

Dinner: 1 serving No-Noodle Eggplant Lasagna with 2 cups mixed greens topped with 1 Tbsp. Herb Vinaigrette (364 calories)

Meal-Prep Tip: Reserve 1 serving of the No-Noodle Eggplant Lasagna to have for lunch tomorrow.

Daily Totals: 1,206 calories, 74 g protein, 103 g carbohydrates, 31 g fiber, 58 g fat, 1,272 mg sodium.

Day 13

Breakfast: 1 serving Muesli with Raspberries (287 calories)

A.M. Snack: 1 large peach (68 calories)

Lunch: 1 serving No-Noodle Eggplant Lasagna (301 calories)

P.M. Snack: 1 cup sliced red bell pepper with 3 Tbsp. hummus (106 calories)

Dinner: 1 serving Slow-Cooker Mediterranean Chicken & Chickpea Soup (446 calories)

Meal-Prep Tip: Reserve 2 servings of the Slow-Cooker Mediterranean Chicken & Chickpea Soup to have for lunch on Days 14 and 15.

Daily Totals: 1,209 calories, 77 g protein, 143 g carbohydrates, 38 g fiber, 40 g fat, 1,431 mg sodium.

Day 14

Breakfast: 1 serving Everything Bagel Avocado Toast with a side of 1 hard-boiled egg (250 calories)

A.M. Snack: 1/2 cup raspberries (31 calories)

Lunch: 1 serving Slow-Cooker Mediterranean Chicken & Chickpea Soup (446 calories)

P.M. Snack: 1/2 cup sliced cucumber with a pinch of salt & pepper (8 calories)

Dinner: 1 serving One-Pot Greek Pasta (487 calories)

Meal-Prep Tip: Prepare 1 serving of Creamy Blueberry-Pecan Overnight Oatmeal so it's ready for breakfast tomorrow.

Daily Totals: 1,224 calories, 69 g protein, 130 g carbohydrates, 30 g fiber, 51 g fat, 1,846 mg sodium.

WEEK 3

Day 15

Breakfast: 1 serving Creamy Blueberry-Pecan Overnight Oatmeal (291 calories)

A.M. Snack: 1 cup blackberries (62 calories)

Lunch: 1 serving Slow-Cooker Mediterranean Chicken & Chickpea Soup (446 calories)

P.M. Snack: 1 plum (30 calories)

Dinner: 1 serving Summer Shrimp Salad with 2 cups mixed greens topped with 1 Tbsp. Parsley-Lemon Vinaigrette (394 calories)

Daily Totals: 1,224 calories, 77 g protein, 127 g carbohydrates, 31 g fiber, 49 g fat, 1,420 mg sodium.

Day 16

Breakfast: 1 serving Muesli with Raspberries (287 calories)

A.M. Snack: 1/2 cup sliced cucumbers with a pinch of salt & pepper (8 calories)

Lunch: 1 serving Vegan Superfood Buddha Bowls (381 calories)

P.M. Snack: 1/2 cup sliced red bell pepper (14 calories)

Dinner: 1 serving Lemon Tahini Couscous with Chicken & Vegetables (528 calories)

Daily Totals: 1,219 calories, 70 g protein, 141 g carbohydrates, 36 g fiber, 49 g fat, 983 mg sodium.

Day 17

Breakfast: 1 serving Muffin-Tin Quiches with Smoked Cheddar & Potato (238 calories)

A.M. Snack: 1/2 cup raspberries (32 calories)

Lunch: 1 serving Vegan Superfood Buddha Bowl (381 calories)

P.M. Snack: 1/2 cup blackberries (31 calories)

Dinner: 1 serving Walnut-Rosemary Crusted Salmon with 1 serving Easy Brown Rice Pilaf with Spring Vegetables (538 calories)

Daily Totals: 1,219 calories, 65 g protein, 120 g carbohydrates, 30 g fiber, 56 g fat, 1,273 mg sodium.

Day 18

Breakfast: 2 servings Berry-Mint Kefir Smoothies (274 calories)

A.M. Snack: 1 plum (30 calories)

Lunch: 1 serving Vegan Superfood Buddha Bowl (381 calories)

P.M. Snack: 1/2 cup nonfat plain Greek yogurt (66 calories)

Dinner: 1 serving Farfalle with Tuna, Lemon & Fennel with 2 cups mixed greens & 1 Tbsp. Parsley-Lemon Vinaigrette (460 calories)

Daily Totals: 1,211 calories, 59 g protein, 155 g carbohydrates, 34 g fiber, 45 g fat, 910 mg sodium.

Day 19

Breakfast: 1 serving Muffin-Tin Quiches with Smoked Cheddar & Potato (238 calories)

A.M. Snack: 1 plum (30 calories)

Lunch: 1 serving Vegan Superfood Buddha Bowls (381 calories)

P.M. Snack: 5 oz. nonfat plain Greek yogurt with 1/4 cup blueberries (105 calories)

Dinner: 1 serving Cilantro Bean Burgers with Creamy Avocado-Lime Slaw with 2 cups mixed greens and 1 Tbsp. Parsley-Lemon Vinaigrette (472 calories)

Daily Totals: 1,226 calories, 63 g protein, 130 g carbohydrates, 34 g fiber, 56 g fat, 1,619 mg sodium.

Day 20

Breakfast: 2 servings Berry-Mint Kefir Smoothies (274 calories)

A.M. Snack: 2/3 cup raspberries (42 calories)

Lunch: 1 serving Mason Jar Power Salad with Chickpeas & Tuna (430 calories)

P.M. Snack: 2/3 cup blackberries (41 calories)

Dinner: 1 serving Roasted Chicken & Winter Squash over Mixed Greens (415 calories)

Daily Totals: 1,202 calories, 72 g protein, 142 g carbohydrates, 34 g fiber, 42 g fat, 1,192 mg sodium.

Day 21

Breakfast: 2 servings Berry-Mint Kefir Smoothies (274 calories)

A.M. Snack: 1/2 cup raspberries (32 calories)

Lunch: 1 serving Mason Jar Power Salad with Chickpeas & Tuna (430 calories)

P.M. Snack: 1/2 cup blackberries (31 calories)

Dinner: 1 serving Sweet & Spicy Roasted Salmon with Wild Rice Pilaf with 2 cups mixed greens and 1 Tbsp. Parsley-Lemon Vinaigrette (443 calories)

Meal-Prep Tip: Reserve 1 serving of the Sweet & Spicy Roasted Salmon with Wild Rice Pilaf to have for lunch tomorrow.

Daily Totals: 1,210 calories, 72 g protein, 145 g carbohydrates, 30 g fiber, 40 g fat, 1,241 mg sodium.

WEEK 4

Day 22

Breakfast: 1 serving Pineapple Green Smoothie (297 calories)

A.M. Snack: 1 cup blackberries (62 calories)

Lunch: 1 salmon fillet (left over from Sweet & Spicy Roasted Salmon with Wild Rice Pilaf) with 1 cup Roasted Butternut Squash & Root Vegetables and 1/3 cup Lemon-Roasted Mixed Vegetables (354 calories)

P.M. Snack: 1 large peach (68 calories)

Dinner: 1 serving Green Salad with Edamame & Beets topped with 1/4 of an avocado (405 calories)

Meal-Prep Tip: Thaw the Slow-Cooker Pasta e Fagioli Soup Freezer Pack in the fridge overnight. Place in the slow cooker tomorrow morning so it's ready in time for dinner.

Daily Totals: 1,187 calories, 63 g protein, 151 g carbohydrates, 44 g fiber, 42 g fat, 1,354 mg sodium.

Day 23

Meal-Prep Tip: Start cooking the Slow-Cooker Pasta e Fagioli Soup Freezer Pack in the morning so it's ready in time for dinner.

Breakfast: 1 serving (287 calories)

A.M. Snack: 1 plum (30 calories)

Lunch: 1 serving Piled-High Greek Vegetable Pitas (399 calories)

P.M. Snack: 1 cup sliced red bell pepper (29 calories)

Dinner: 1 serving Slow-Cooker Pasta e Fagioli Soup Freezer Pack (457 calories)

Daily Totals: 1,202 calories, 63 g protein, 160 g carbohydrates, 36 g fiber, 40 g fat, 1,461 mg sodium.

Day 24

Breakfast: 1 serving Everything Bagel Avocado Toast with a side of 1 hard-boiled egg (250 calories)

A.M. Snack: 2/3 cup raspberries (42 calories)

Lunch: 1 serving Piled-High Greek Vegetable Pitas (399 calories)

P.M. Snack: 1 plum (30 calories)

Dinner: 1 serving Quinoa, Chicken & Broccoli Salad with Roasted Lemon Dressing (481 calories)

Meal-Prep Tip: Prepare the Blueberry Almond Chia Pudding to have for breakfast tomorrow.

Daily Totals: 1,202 calories, 50 g protein, 131 g carbohydrates, 33 g fiber, 57 g fat, 1,403 mg sodium.

Day 25

Breakfast: 1 serving Blueberry Almond Chia Pudding (229 calories)

A.M. Snack: 5 oz. nonfat plain Greek yogurt with 1/4 cup blueberries and 1 Tbsp. chopped walnuts (153 calories)

Lunch: 1 serving Piled-High Greek Vegetable Pitas (399 calories)

P.M. Snack: 1 large peach (68 calories)

Dinner: 1 serving Mediterranean Cod with Roasted Tomatoes and 3/4 cup Quinoa Avocado Salad (364 calories)

Daily Totals: 1,213 calories, 65 g protein, 140 g carbohydrates, 35 g fiber, 49 g fat, 1,450 mg sodium.

Day 26

Breakfast: 1 serving Everything Bagel Avocado Toast with a side of 1 hard-boiled egg (250 calories)

A.M. Snack: 1 cup raspberries (64 calories)

Lunch: 1 serving Piled-High Greek Vegetable Pitas (399 calories)

P.M. Snack: 5 oz. nonfat plain Greek yogurt with 1/3 cup blackberries (104 calories)

Dinner: serving Caprese Stuffed Portobello Mushrooms with 3/4 cup Quinoa Avocado Salad (393 calories)

Meal-Prep Tip: Transfer 4 servings of the Instant Pot White Chicken Chili Freezer Pack to the fridge to defrost for lunch on Days 27, 28, 29 and 30.

Daily Totals: 1,210 calories, 54 g protein, 124 g carbohydrates, 37 g fiber, 60 g fat, 1,559 mg sodium.

Day 27

Breakfast: 1 serving Muesli with Raspberries (287 calories)

A.M. Snack: 1 large peach (68 calories)

Lunch: 1 serving Instant Pot White Chicken Chili Freezer Pack with 1/2 cup blueberries (298 calories)

P.M. Snack: 3/4 cup sliced red bell pepper with 1 Tbsp. hummus (47 calories)

Dinner: 1 serving Stuffed Eggplant with 1 serving Traditional Greek Salad (513 calories)

Daily Totals: 1,214 calories, 54 g protein, 157 g carbohydrates, 39 g fiber, 49 g fat, 1,739 mg sodium.

Day 28

Breakfast: 2 servings Berry-Mint Kefir Smoothies (274 calories)

A.M. Snack: 1/2 cup sliced red bell pepper (14 calories)

Lunch: 1 serving Instant Pot White Chicken Chili Freezer Pack with 1/2 cup blueberries (298 calories)

P.M. Snack: 1/2 cup sliced cucumbers with a pinch of salt & pepper (8 calories)

Dinner: 1 serving Chickpea Pasta with Lemony-Parsley Pesto (630 calories)

Daily Totals: 1,224 calories, 53 g protein, 154 g carbohydrates, 33 g fiber, 50 g fat, 1,491 mg sodium.

WEEK 5

Day 29

Breakfast: 1 serving Everything Bagel Avocado Toast with a side of 1 hard-boiled egg (250 calories)

A.M. Snack: 2/3 cup fresh raspberries with 5 walnut halves (108 calories)

Lunch: 1 serving Instant Pot White Chicken Chili Freezer Pack with 1/2 cup blueberries (298 calories)

P.M. Snack: 2/3 cup blackberries with 7 walnut halves (132 calories)

Dinner: 1 serving Greek Roasted Fish with Vegetables (422 calories)

Daily Totals: 1,210 calories, 74 g protein, 119 g carbohydrates, 35 g fiber, 53 g fat, 1,613 mg sodium.

Lunch: 1 serving Instant Pot White Chicken Chili Freezer Pack with 1/2 cup blueberries (298 calories)

P.M. Snack: 12 walnut halves (157 calories)

Dinner: 1 serving Slow-Cooker Mediterranean Chicken & Orzo with 1 serving Cucumber, Tomato & Avocado Salad (450 calories)

Daily Totals: 1,201 calories, 66 g protein, 138 g carbohydrates, 38 g fiber, 49 g fat, 1,537 mg sodium.

Day 30

Breakfast: 1 serving Blueberry Almond Chia Pudding (229 calories)

A.M. Snack: 1 large peach (68 calories)

LET'S START!
MEDITERRANEAN RECIPES

MEDITERRANEAN BREAKFAST RECIPE

Creamy Paninis

Total time: 15 minutes

Prep time: 10 minutes

Cook time: 5 minutes

Yield: 4 servings

Ingredients

- 2 tbsp. finely chopped black olives, oil-cured
- ¼ cup chopped fresh basil leaves
- ½ cup mayonnaise dressing with Olive Oil, divided
- 8 slices whole-wheat bread
- 4 slices of bacon
- 1 small zucchini, thinly sliced
- 4 slices provolone cheese
- 7 oz. roasted red peppers, sliced

Directions

- In a small bowl, combine olives, basil, and ¼ cup of mayonnaise; evenly spread the mayonnaise mixture on the bread slices and layer 4 slices with bacon, zucchini, provolone and peppers.
- Top with the remaining bread slices and spread the remaining ¼ cup of mayonnaise on the outside of the sandwiches; cook over medium heat for about 4 minutes, turning once, until cheese is melted and the sandwiches are golden brown.

Breakfast Couscous

Total time: 15 minutes

Prep time: 10 minutes

Cook time: 5 minutes

Yield: 4 servings

Ingredients

- 1 (2-inch) cinnamon stick
- 3 cups 1% low-fat milk
- 1 cup whole-wheat couscous (uncooked)
- 6 tsp. dark brown sugar, divided
- ¼ cup dried currants
- ½ cup chopped apricots (dried)
- ¼ tsp. sea salt
- 4 tsp. melted butter, divided

Directions

- In a saucepan set over medium high heat, combine cinnamon stick and milk; heat for about 3 minutes (do not boil).
- Remove the pan from heat and stir in couscous, 4 teaspoons of sugar, currants, apricots, and sea salt. Let the mixture stand, covered, for at least 15 minutes.
- Discard the cinnamon stick and divide the couscous among four bowls; top each serving with ½ teaspoon of sugar and 1 teaspoon of melted butter. Serve immediately.

Potato and Chickpea Hash

Total time: 15 minutes

Prep time: 10 minutes

Cook time: 5 minutes

Yield: 4 servings

Ingredients

- 4 cups shredded frozen hash brown potatoes
- 1 tbsp. freshly minced ginger

- ½ cup chopped onion
- 2 cups chopped baby spinach
- 1 tbsp. curry powder
- ½ tsp. sea salt
- ¼ cup extra virgin olive oil
- 1 cup chopped zucchini
- 1 (15-ounce) can chickpeas, rinsed
- 4 large eggs

Directions

- In a large bowl, combine the potatoes, ginger, onion, spinach, curry powder, and sea salt.
- In a nonstick skillet set over medium high heat, heat extra virgin olive oil and add the potato mixture.
- Press the mixture into a layer and cook for about 5 minutes, without stirring, or until golden brown and crispy.
- Lower heat to medium low and fold in zucchini and chickpeas, breaking up the mixture until just combined.
- Stir briefly, press the mixture back into a layer, and make four wells.
- Break one egg into each indentation.
- Cook, covered, for about 5 minutes or until eggs are set.

Avocado Toast

Total time: 10 minutes

Prep time: 10 minutes

Cook time: 0 minutes

Yield: 4 servings

Ingredients

- 2 ripe avocados, peeled
- Squeeze of fresh lemon juice, to taste

- 2 tbsp. freshly chopped mint, plus extra to garnish
- Sea salt and black pepper, to taste
- 4 large slices rye bread
- 80 grams soft feta, crumbled

Directions

- In a medium bowl, mash the avocado roughly with a fork; add lemon juice and mint and continue mashing until just combined.
- Season with black pepper and sea salt to taste.
- Grill or toast bread until golden.
- Spread about ¼ of the avocado mixture onto each slice of the toasted bread and top with feta.
- Garnish with extra mint and serve immediately.

Mediterranean Pancakes

Total time: 50 minutes

Prep time: 30 minutes

Cook time: 20 minutes

Yield: 16 Pancakes

Ingredients

- 1 cup old-fashioned oats
- ½ cup all-purpose flour
- 2 tbsp. flax seeds
- 1 tsp. baking soda
- ¼ tsp. sea salt
- 2 tbsp. extra virgin olive oil
- 2 large eggs
- 2 cups nonfat plain Greek yogurt
- 2 tbsp. raw honey
- Fresh fruit, syrup, or other toppings

Directions

- In a blender, combine oats, flour, flax seeds, baking soda, and sea salt; blend for about 30 seconds.
- Add extra virgin olive oil, eggs, yogurt, and honey and continue pulsing until very smooth.
- Let the mixture stand for at least 20 minutes or until thick.
- Set a large nonstick skillet over medium heat and brush with extra virgin olive oil.
- In batches, ladle the batter by quarter-cupfuls into the skillet.
- Cook the pancakes for about 2 minutes or until bubbles form and golden brown.
- Turn them over and cook the other sides for 2 minutes more or until golden brown.
- Transfer the cooked pancakes to a baking sheet and keep warm in oven.
- Serve with favorite toppings.

Mediterranean Frittata

Total time: 25 minutes

Prep time: 10 minutes

Cook time: 15 minutes

Yield: 4 servings

Ingredients

- 3 tbsp. extra virgin olive oil, divided
- 1 cup chopped onion
- 2 cloves garlic, minced
- 8 eggs, beaten
- ¼ cup half-and-half, milk or light cream
- ½ cup sliced Kalamata olives
- ½ cup roasted red sweet peppers, chopped
- ½ cup crumbled feta cheese
- ⅛ tsp. black pepper
- ¼ cup fresh basil
- 2 tbsp. Parmesan cheese, finely shredded
- ½ cup coarsely crushed onion-and-garlic croutons
- Fresh basil leaves, to garnish

Directions

- Preheat your broiler.
- Heat 2 tablespoons of extra virgin olive oil in a broiler-proof skillet set over medium heat; sauté onion and garlic for a few minutes or until tender.
- In the meantime, beat eggs and half-and-half in a bowl until well combined.
- Stir in olives, roasted sweet pepper, feta cheese, black pepper and basil.
- Pour the egg mixture over the sautéed onion mixture and cook until almost set.
- With a spatula, lift the egg mixture to allow the uncooked part to flow underneath.
- Continue cooking for 2 minutes more or until the set.
- Combine the remaining extra virgin olive oil, Parmesan cheese, and crushed croutons in a bowl; sprinkle the mixture over the frittata and broil for about 5 minutes or until the crumbs are golden and the top is set.
- To serve, cut the frittata into wedges and garnish with fresh basil.

Nutty Banana Oatmeal

Total time: 15 minutes

Prep time: 10 minutes

Cook time: 5 minutes

Yield: 4 servings

Ingredients

- ¼ cup quick cooking oats
- 3 tbsp. raw honey
- ½ cup skim milk
- 2 tbsp. chopped walnuts
- 1 tsp. flax seeds
- 1 banana, peeled

Directions

- In a microwave-safe bowl, combine oats, honey, milk, walnuts, and flaxseeds; microwave on high for about 2 minutes.
- In a small bowl, mash the banana with a fork to a fine consistency; stir into the oatmeal and serve hot.

Mediterranean Veggie Omelet

Total time: 40 minutes

Prep time: 15 minutes

Cook time: 25 minutes

Yield: 4 servings

Ingredients

- 1 tbsp. extra virgin olive oil
- 2 cups thinly sliced fresh fennel bulb
- ¼ cup chopped artichoke hearts, soaked in water, drained
- ¼ cup pitted green olives, brine-cured, chopped
- 1 diced Roma tomato
- 6 eggs
- ¼ tsp. sea salt
- ½ tsp. freshly ground black pepper
- ½ cup goat cheese, crumbled
- 2 tbsp. freshly chopped fresh parsley, dill, or basil

Directions

- Preheat your oven to 325°F.
- Heat extra virgin olive oil in an ovenproof skillet over medium heat.
- Sauté fennel for about 5 minutes or until tender.
- Add artichoke hearts, olives, and tomatoes and cook for 3minutes ore or until softened.
- In a bowl, beat the eggs; season with sea salt and pepper.
- Add the egg mixture over the vegetables and stir for about 2 minutes.
- Sprinkle cheese over the omelet and bake in the oven for about 5 minutes or until set and cooked through.
- Top with parsley, dill, or basil.
- Transfer the omelet onto a cutting board, carefully cut into four wedges, and serve immediately.

Lemon Scones

Total time: 30 minutes

Prep time: 15 minutes

Cook time: 15 minutes

Yield: 12 servings

Ingredients

- 2 cups plus ¼ cup flour
- ½ tsp. baking soda
- 2 tbsp. sugar

- ½ tsp. sea salt
- ¾ cup reduced-fat buttermilk
- Zest of 1 lemon
- 1 to 2 tsp. freshly squeezed lemon juice
- 1 cup powdered sugar

Directions

- Preheat your oven to 400°F.
- In a food processor, combine 2 cups of flour, baking soda, sugar and salt until well blended.
- Add buttermilk and lemon zest and continue mixing to combine well.
- Sprinkle the remaining flour onto a clean surface and turn out the dough; gently knead the dough at least six times and shape it into a ball.
- Using a rolling pin, flatten the dough into half-inch thick circle.
- Cut the dough into four equal wedges and the cut each into three smaller wedges.
- Arrange the scones on a baking sheet and bake in preheated oven for about 15 minutes or until golden brown.
- Mix together lemon juice and the powdered sugar in a small bowl to make a thin frosting.
- Remove the scones from the oven and drizzle with lemon frosting while still hot.
- Serve right away.

Breakfast Wrap

Total time: 10 minutes

Prep time: 5 minutes

Cooking time: 5 minutes

Yield: 2 servings

Ingredients

- ½ cup fresh-picked spinach
- 4 egg whites
- 2 Bella sun-dried tomatoes
- 2 mixed-grain flax wraps
- ½ cup feta cheese crumbles

Directions

- Cook spinach, egg whites and tomatoes in a frying pan for about 4 minutes or until lightly browned.
- Flip it over and cook the other side for 4 minutes or until almost done.
- Microwave the wraps for about 15 seconds; remove from the microwave, fill each wrap with the egg mixture, sprinkle with feta cheese crumbles and roll up.
- Cut each wrap into two parts and serve.

Garlicky Scrambled Eggs

Total time: 25 minutes

Prep time: 10 minutes

Cooking time: 15 minutes

Yield: 2 servings

Ingredients

- ½ tsp. extra virgin olive oil
- ½ cup ground beef
- ½ tsp. garlic powder
- 3 eggs
- Salt
- Pepper

Directions

- Set a medium-sized pan over medium heat.

- Add extra virgin olive oil and heat until hot but not smoking.
- Stir in ground beef and cook for about 10 minutes or until almost done.
- Stir in garlic and sauté for about 2 minutes.
- In a large bowl, beat the eggs until almost frothy; season with salt and pepper.
- Add the egg mixture to the pan with the cooked beef and scramble until ready.
- Serve with toasted bread and olives, for a healthy, satisfying breakfast!

Healthy Breakfast Casserole

Total time: 60 minutes

Prep time: 10 minutes

Cooking time: 50 minutes

Yield: 6 servings

Ingredients

- 2 tbsp. extra virgin olive oil, divided
- ½ a medium-sized onion, diced
- 2 medium-sized yellow potatoes. diced
- 1 lb. zucchini, sliced
- 3 portabella mushroom caps, diced
- 150g torn fresh spinach
- 200g ricotta
- 200g light ricotta cheese
- 2 cups of egg whites
- 12 grape tomatoes,sliced into⅓ pieces
- 3 peeled and roasted fresh peppers, sliced
- 2 sourdough rolls
- 4 tbsp. Pecorino Romano cheese, grated
- 100g skim-milk mozzarella cheese, grated

Directions

- Preheat the oven to 400°F.
- Mix together olive oil, onion and potato and roast for at least 15 minutes; remove from oven and keep on the baking tray.
- In a bowl, combine together ½ tablespoon olive oil and zucchini; toss to coat well and transfer to a baking tray.
- Return all the vegetables to oven and roast for about 40 minutes or until golden in color.
- In the meantime, place ½ tablespoon olive oil in a pan and sauté mushrooms for about 4 minutes.
- Remove the cooked mushrooms from pan and set aside.
- Add the remaining olive oil to pan and sauté chopped spinach until tender.
- In a mixing bowl, combine together both types of ricotta and egg whites; set aside.
- Combine together all the vegetables, including grape tomatoes and peppers, with sourdough rolls in a 9 x 13 baking dish; top with the ricotta mixture and sprinkle with pecorino and mozzarella cheese.
- Bake for at least 40 minutes or until done. Remove from the oven, cool slightly.
- Cut into six slices and enjoy your breakfast.

Egg and Sausage Breakfast Casserole

Total time: 1 hour, 25 minutes

Prep time: 20 minutes

Cook time: 1 hour, 5 minutes

Yield: 12 servings

Ingredients

The crust:

- 3 tbsp. olive oil, divided
- 2 lb. peeled and shredded russet potatoes
- ¾ tsp. ground pepper
- ¾ tsp. salt

The casserole:

- 12 oz. chopped turkey sausage
- 4 thinly sliced green onions
- ¼ cup diced bell pepper
- ⅓ cup skim milk
- 6 large eggs
- 4 egg whites
- ¾ cup shredded cheddar cheese
- 16 oz. low-fat cottage cheese

Directions

The crust:

- Preheat the oven to 425°F. Lightly grease a 9×13-inch baking dish with 1 tbsp. olive oil and set aside.
- Squeeze excess moisture out of the potato with a kitchen towel or paper towel.
- Toss together the potatoes, the remaining olive oil, salt and pepper in a medium bowl until potatoes are well coated.

- Transfer the mixture to the greased baking dish; evenly press the mixture up the sides and on the bottom of the dish and bake for about 20 minutes or until golden brown on the edges.

The casserole:

- Reduce the oven heat to 375°F.
- In a large skillet, cook turkey sausage over medium-high heat for about 2 minutes or until it's almost cooked through.
- Add green onions and red bell pepper and continue cooking for 2 more minutes or until bell pepper is tender.
- Whisk together skim milk, eggs, egg whites, and the cheeses.
- Stir in turkey sausage mixture; pour over the potato crust and bake for about 50 minutes. Slightly cool and cut into 12 pieces. Enjoy!

Yogurt Pancakes

Total time: 15 minutes

Prep time: 10 minutes

Cooking time: 5 minutes

Yield: 5 servings

Ingredients

- Whole-wheat pancake mix
- 1 cup yogurt
- 1 tbsp. baking powder
- 1 tbsp. baking soda
- 1 cup skimmed milk
- 3 whole eggs
- ½ tsp. extra virgin olive oil

Directions

- Combine together whole-wheat pancake mix, yogurt, baking powder, baking soda, skimmed milk and eggs in large bowl.
- Stir until well blended.
- Heat a pan oiled lightly with olive oil.
- Pour ¼ cup batter onto the heated pan and cook for about 2 minutes or until the surface of the pancake has some bubbles.
- Flip and continue cooking until the underside is browned.
- Serve the pancakes warm with a cup of fat-free milk or two tablespoons light maple syrup.

Breakfast Stir Fry

Total time: 25 minutes
Prep time: 5 minutes
Cooking time: 20 minutes
Yield: 4 servings

Ingredients

- 1 tbsp. extra virgin olive oil
- 2 green peppers, sliced
- 2 small onions, finely chopped
- 4 tomatoes, chopped
- ½ tsp. sea salt
- 1 egg

Directions

- Heat olive oil in a medium-sized pan over medium-high heat.
- Add green pepper and sauté for about 2 minutes.
- Lower heat to medium and continue cooking, covered, for 3 more minutes.

- Stir in onion and cook for about 2 minutes or until brown.
- Stir in tomatoes and salt; cover and simmer to get a soft juicy mixture.
- In a bowl, beat the egg; drizzle over the tomato mixture and cook for about 1 minute. (Don't stir).
- Serve with chopped cucumbers, feta cheese and black olives for a great breakfast!

Greek Breakfast Pitas

Total time: 20 minutes
Prep time: 10 minutes
Cook time: 10 minutes
Yield: 4 servings

Ingredients

- ¼ cup chopped onion
- ¼ cup sweet red/black pepper, chopped
- 1 cup large egg
- ⅛ tsp. sea salt
- ⅛ tsp. black pepper
- 1 ½ tsp. fresh basil, ground
- ½ cup baby spinach, freshly torn
- 1 red tomato, sliced
- 2 pita bread, whole
- 2 tbsp. feta cheese, crumbled

Directions

- Coat a sizeable nonstick skillet with cooking spray and set over medium heat.
- Add onions and red peppers and sauté for at least 3 minutes.
- In a small bowl, beat together egg, pepper and salt and add the mixture to the skillet.

- Cook, stirring continuously, until ready.
- Spoon basil, spinach, and tomatoes onto the pitas and top with the egg mixture.
- Sprinkle with feta and serve.

Healthy Breakfast Scramble

Total time: 20 minutes

Prep time: 5 minutes

Cook time: 15 minutes

Yield: 2 servings

Ingredients

- 1 tsp. extra virgin olive
- 4 medium green onions, chopped
- 1 tsp. dried basil leaves or 1 tbsp. fresh basil leaves, chopped
- 1 medium tomato, chopped
- 4 eggs
- Freshly ground pepper

Directions

- In a medium nonstick skillet, heat olive oil over medium heat; sauté green onions, stirring occasionally, for about 2 minutes.
- Stir in basil and tomato and let cook, stirring occasionally, for about 1 minute or until the tomato is cooked through.
- In a small bowl, thoroughly beat the eggs with a wire whisk or a fork and pour over the tomato mixture; cook for about 2 minutes.
- Gently lift the cooked parts with spatula to allow the uncooked parts to flow to the bottom.
- Continue cooking for about 3 minutes or until the eggs are cooked through.

- Season with pepper and serve.

Greek Parfait

Total time: 6 minutes

Prep time: 6 minutes

Cook time: 0 minutes

Yield: 6 servings

Ingredients

- 1 tsp. vanilla extract
- 3 cups low-fat Greek yogurt
- ¼ cup toasted unsalted pistachios, shelled
- 4 tsp. raw honey
- 28 Clementine segments

Directions

- In a mixing bowl, combine the vanilla extract with the Greek yogurt.
- Spoon ¼ cup of the mixture into 4 small parfait glasses.
- Top each of the 4 glasses with ½ tablespoon nuts, ½ teaspoon honey and 5 Clementine sections.
- Add the remaining yogurt mixture to the parfait glasses and top with ½ tablespoon nuts, Clementine segments and ½ teaspoon honey.
- Serve immediately

Quiche Wrapped in Prosciutto

Total time: 25 minutes

Prep time: 10 minutes

Cook time: 15 minutes

Yield: 8 servings

Ingredients

- 4 slices prosciutto, halved

- 2 egg whites
- 1 egg
- ½ tsp. rosemary, fresh and chopped and a little more for garnishing
- 3tbsp. low fat Greek yoghurt
- 1 tbsp. chopped black olives
- A pinch of black pepper, freshly ground
  A pinch of salt

Directions

- Preheat your oven to 400°F and coat your muffin baking tray with cooking spray.
- Place each prosciutto piece into eight cups of the tray.
- In a medium bowl, whisk the egg whites and the egg until smooth.
- Pour in the yogurt, rosemary, olives, pepper, and salt and continue whisking.
- Divide the mixture equally among the prosciutto cups and bake uncovered until cooked through (about 15 minutes).
- Garnish with rosemary.

Morning Couscous

Total time: 35 minutes

Prep time 10 minutes

Cook time 25 minutes

Yield: 4 servings

Ingredients

- 3 cups soy milk
- 1 cinnamon stick
- 1 cup whole-wheat couscous, uncooked
- ¼ cup currants, dried
- ½ cup apricots, dried
- 4 tsp. sun butter, melted and divided
- 6 tsp. brown sugar, divided
- 1 pinch salt

Directions

- Put a saucepan on medium heat and pour in soy milk and the cinnamon stick.
- Let it heat for 3 minutes or until tiny bubbles start forming on the inner part of the pan; do not let it boil.
- Remove the saucepan from the heat and stir in the couscous, currants, apricots, salt, and 4 tablespoons of sugar.
- Put a lid on the pan and let it stand for 20 minutes. Remove the cinnamon stick.
- Divide the couscous among 4 bowls and top with ½ teaspoon of sugar and 1 teaspoon melted sun butter.
- Serve hot.

Green Omelet

Total time: 15 minutes

Prep time: 5 minutes

Cook time: 10 minutes

Yield: 4 servings

Ingredients

- 8 eggs
- 1 yellow onion, finely chopped
- 1 clove garlic, minced
- 1 medium bunch of collard greens
- 3 tbsp. parsley, chopped
- 1 tsp. allspice
- 5 tbsp. extra virgin olive oil
- ½ cup Parmigiano-Reggiano cheese, grated   1 pinch sea salt, optional

Directions

- Beat the eggs in a big bowl and add the onion, garlic, collard greens, parsley, and allspice.
- Continue beating until all the ingredients mix well.
- Put a nonstick skillet on medium heat and pour in the olive oil until hot.
- Add the contents of the bowl and let cook for about 5 minutes or until it turns golden brown.
- Use a spatula to flip the omelet and cook the other side for 5 minutes or until it turns golden brown.
- Serve on a plate, cut into desired portions, then sprinkle the grated cheese and you are ready to eat.

Healthy Quinoa

Total time: 25 minutes

Prep time: 10 minutes

Cook time: 15 minutes

Yield: 4 servings

Ingredients

- 1 cup almonds
- 1 tsp. ground cinnamon
- 1 cup quinoa
- 2 cups milk
- 1 pinch sea salt
- 2 tbsp. honey
- 5 dried apricots, finely chopped
- 2 dried, pitted dates, finely chopped
- 1 tsp. vanilla extract

Directions

- Start by toasting the almonds on a skillet for five minutes or until golden brown for a good nutty flavor.
- Place a saucepan over medium heat and add the quinoa and cinnamon; heat until warmed through.
- Follow by adding the milk and sea salt while stirring all along.
- Once the mixture comes to a boil, reduce the heat, cover the saucepan and let it simmer for 15 minutes.
- Add the honey, apricots, dates, vanilla extract and half the almonds into the saucepan.
- Serve in bowls and top with the remaining almonds.

MUSHROOM STRAPATSATHA WITH

HALLOUMI AND CRISPY BACON

There are so many mushroom varieties. Be creative and mix them up in this recipe.

Serves 4

- 1/4 cup plus 2 tablespoons extra-virgin olive oil, divided 1/3 cup chopped onions or scallions 1 clove garlic, peeled and minced
- 1 cup sliced cremini mushrooms
- 1 teaspoon salt, divided
- 1/2 teaspoon pepper, divided 1 cup sliced oyster mushrooms
- 4 (1/4-inch) slices halloumi cheese, roughly chopped 8 large eggs, beaten
- 1/4 cup heavy cream or evaporated milk 1 teaspoon fresh thyme leaves
- 1 teaspoon chopped fresh tarragon
- 4 strips crispy cooked bacon, crumbled and divided
- 2 tablespoons chopped fresh chives
- 1 cup jarred or homemade salsa

Directions

- In a large skillet over medium heat, add 1/4 cup oil and heat for 30 seconds. Add onions and garlic and cook for 5 minutes or until onions are softened. Add cremini mushrooms and season with 1/2 teaspoon salt and 1/4 teaspoon pepper. Cook for 5 minutes or until the mushrooms are lightly browned. Add the oyster mushrooms and cook for 2 minutes. Stir in the halloumi and cook for 1 more minute.
- In a medium bowl, whisk together eggs, cream or milk, thyme, tarragon, and the remaining salt and pepper. Add the eggs to the mushrooms and stir until the eggs are scrambled. Stir in bacon.

- Serve topped with chives and salsa. Drizzle with remaining oil and serve immediately.

BREAKFAST BAKLAVA FRENCH TOAST

Use day-old bread like challah or Tsoureki (Greek Easter Bread) (see recipe in Chapter 3) to make this French toast.

Serves 2

- 3 large eggs
- 2 tablespoons orange juice
- 1 teaspoon grated orange zest
- 1/8 teaspoon vanilla extract 1/4 cup plus 1 tablespoon honey, divided 2 tablespoons whole milk
- 1 1/4 teaspoons ground cinnamon, divided 1/4 cup walnuts
- 1/4 cup blanched almonds
- 1/4 teaspoon ground cloves
- 1 tablespoon sugar
- 2 tablespoons white bread crumbs or ground melba toast 4 slices bread
- 2 tablespoons unsalted butter
- 1 teaspoon confectioners' sugar

Directions

- In a large bowl, whisk together eggs, orange juice, zest, vanilla, 1/4 cup honey, milk, and 1/2 teaspoon cinnamon. Reserve.
- Put the walnuts and almonds into a food processor, and pulse until they are finely crumbled. Transfer the nuts to a bowl and add the cloves, 1/2 teaspoon

cinnamon, sugar, and bread crumbs. Stir to combine.

- Sandwich half of the walnut-and-almond mixture between 2 slices of bread. Repeat with the remaining 2 slices. Carefully dunk both sides of the sandwiches into the egg mixture. Make sure the egg mixture soaks into the bread.
- Add the butter to a large skillet over medium heat, and heat for 30 seconds. Add the sandwiches and fry for 2 minutes per side or until golden.
- Carefully cut the French toasts diagonally and serve them dusted with confectioners' sugar.
- Drizzle the tops with the remaining honey and sprinkle with 1/4 teaspoon cinnamon. Serve immediately.

TIGANITES

Tiganites is the Greek equivalent of pancakes. Instead of maple syrup, drizzle with honey or petimezi, a grape molasses found in Greek, Turkish, and Middle Eastern shops.

Serves 4

- 2 cups all-purpose flour
- 2 tablespoons sugar
- 2 teaspoons baking powder
- 3/4 teaspoon salt 2 large eggs
- 2 cups whole milk
- 1/4 cup vegetable oil 4 tablespoons unsalted butter, divided
- 1/4 cup honey or petimezi (grape molasses)

Directions

- In a medium bowl, combine flour, sugar, baking powder, and salt.
- In another medium bowl, whisk together eggs, milk, and oil.
- Add the dry ingredients to the wet ingredients and stir to combine.
- In a large skillet over medium heat, add 2 tablespoons butter and heat for 30 seconds. To make a pancake, pour 1⁄4 cup of batter into the pan. Cook until you see bubbles forming on the top side of the pancake (about 2 minutes), then flip the pancake over and cook for another 2 minutes. Remove the pancake from the pan and keep warm. Repeat with the remaining batter.
- Serve hot topped with remaining butter and honey.

BEET AND WALNUT MUFFINS

Serves 12

- 2 cups plus 1⁄4 cup all-purpose flour, divided 1 tablespoon baking powder
- 3⁄4 cup sugar 1⁄2 teaspoon salt 2 teaspoons ground cinnamon
- 2 large eggs, beaten
- 1 cup whole milk
- 1⁄4 cup extra-virgin olive oil
- 2 cups grated beets, peeled
- 3⁄4 cup chopped walnuts

Directions

- In a medium bowl, combine 2 cups flour, baking powder, sugar, salt, and cinnamon. In another medium bowl, whisk together eggs, milk, and oil.
- In another medium bowl, combine beets, walnuts, and the remaining flour. Toss to combine the ingredients, and to coat the beets and walnuts in flour.
- Preheat the oven to 375°F. Add the wet ingredients to the dry ingredients, and stir to combine. Stir in the walnuts and beets. Don't overmix the batter or the muffins will be tough.
- Line a 12-muffin tin with paper cups and divide the batter evenly among the 12 cups. Bake on the middle rack 15–20 minutes. Stick a toothpick into a muffin; if the toothpick comes out clean, the muffins are done.
- Transfer the muffins to a cooling rack. Allow them to cool before removing them from the pan and serving.

FIG JAM

If you're lucky enough to find ripe figs, try this easy recipe and make some delicious fig jam. Preserving this summer fruit makes the cold months bearable.

Makes 6 cups

- 65–70 medium ripe figs, stems removed and halved
- 2 cups granulated sugar
- 1 cup water
- 2 teaspoons vanilla extract
- 5 fresh basil leaves
- 1 1⁄2 teaspoons grated lemon zest
- 1 tablespoon fresh lemon juice

Directions

- In a large pot over medium-high heat, add figs, sugar, water, and vanilla. Bring the water to a boil, then reduce the heat to medium-low and cook for 45 minutes. Remove the pot from the heat and allow the jam to cool completely (about 4 hours). Mash the figs to the desired consistency— chunky or smooth.
- Return the pot to the stove over low heat for 5 minutes. Add basil leaves and simmer 5–6 minutes. Add the lemon zest and juice and simmer another 5–6 minutes. Take the pot off the heat and remove the basil leaves. Again, let the jam cool completely.
- Pour the jam into sterilized jars and seal them according to standard jarring procedures.

HOMEMADE GREEK YOGURT

Greeks have been making and consuming yogurt for thousands of years. Ignore all the yogurts in the grocery store and make your own.
Makes 16 cups

- 16 cups whole milk
- 1/2 cup plain full-fat yogurt (containing active live cultures)

Directions

- Preheat the oven to 200°F. In a large pot over medium-high heat, add the milk and bring it to a boil. Reduce the heat to medium-low and simmer for 15 minutes, and then take the pot off the heat. Do not cover the pot.

- Using a candy thermometer, allow the milk to cool to 110°F–115°F. When you have reached the desired temperature, combine 1/2 cup of warm milk with yogurt in a small bowl. Stir to combine. Add the milk and yogurt back to the pot and stir to combine.
- Turn off the oven. Ladle the milk-yogurt mixture into storage containers (plastic containers are okay because the oven is at a low temperature) and place on a baking tray in the oven. The yogurt will set in 8–12 hours (check it after 8 hours).
- Refrigerate the yogurt for at least 4 hours, but preferably overnight. This yogurt will keep in the refrigerator for up to 2 weeks.

STRAPATSATHA

Strapatsatha is a dish brought to Greece by the Sephardic Jews from Spain. It's a loose omelet of tomatoes and feta. There are many variations of this classic dish.
Serves 4

- 1/4 cup extra-virgin olive oil
- 2/3 cup sliced chorizo sausage
- 4 large ripe tomatoes, passed through a box grater
- 1/2 cup diced sweet banana pepper
- 3 scallions, ends trimmed and sliced
- 1 cup crumbled feta cheese
- 8 large eggs, beaten
- 1/2 teaspoon pepper

Directions

- Add oil to a large skillet over medium-high heat, and heat for 30 seconds. Add sausage and cook for 2 minutes or until it browns. With a slotted spoon, remove the sausage from the skillet and reserve. Take the skillet off the heat and let it cool for 5 minutes.

- Return the skillet to a medium heat and add the tomatoes. Cook for 5 minutes or until most of the water is evaporated. Add the peppers and scallions, and cook for 2 more minutes. Add the feta and cook for 1 minute.

- Add the eggs, pepper, and cooked sausage. Stir the eggs to scramble them, cooking them until they form a loose omelet. Serve immediately or warm.

CHEESE PIES IN YOGURT PASTRY

These crescent-shaped pies are ideal for family members who are rushed in the morning. They can grab a couple of pies and eat on the go! Serves 10

- 2 large eggs, divided
- 1⁄2 cup extra-virgin olive oil 3⁄4 cup plain yogurt 1 teaspoon salt
- 31⁄2 cups self-rising flour, sifted 1 cup crumbled feta cheese
- 1 cup ricotta cheese
- 1⁄4 cup grated Graviera (or Gruyère) cheese
- 1⁄2 teaspoon grated fresh nutmeg
- 1⁄4 teaspoon pepper
- 1 tablespoon finely chopped fresh mint

- 1 large egg yolk
- 1 tablespoon cream
- 1⁄2 cup sesame seeds

Directions

- In a large bowl, whisk together 1 egg, the oil, and yogurt. Combine the salt and flour in another bowl. Using a wooden spoon, stir the dry ingredients into the wet ingredients to form dough. Transfer the dough onto a work surface and knead it until all the flour is incorporated. The dough should be smooth, pliable, and only slightly sticky. Wrap dough in plastic wrap and set it aside.

- Preheat the oven to 350°F. In a large bowl, combine the remaining egg, the cheeses, nutmeg, pepper, and mint. Mash and mix together with a wooden spoon.

- Place the dough on a lightly floured work surface and roll it out into a long thin log. Cut the dough into egg-size pieces (you should get twenty). Roll a dough piece into a ball and then flatten it with the palm of your hand into a 3-inch-thin disc. Add 1 tablespoon cheese filling in the middle of the dough. Fold half of the dough over the filling to create a crescent shape. Pinch the ends to seal the cheese into the dough. Place the pie on a parchment-lined baking sheet, and repeat the process with the remaining dough and cheese filling.

- In a small bowl, whisk together the egg yolk and cream. Brush the top of each pie with the egg-cream mixture. Sprinkle the tops with sesame seeds.

- Bake the pies on the middle rack for 30 minutes or until they are golden. Serve them warm or at room temperature. You can store pies in a container in the refrigerator for up to 5 days.

PAXIMADIA

Makes 36

- 3 large eggs, beaten
- 1½ cups vegetable oil
- 1½ cups sugar
- 2 teaspoons vanilla extract
- 1 teaspoon almond extract
- 4 cups all-purpose flour
- 1 teaspoon baking powder
- 1 cup chopped almonds
- 1 cup sesame seeds

Directions

- Preheat the oven to 350°F. In a large bowl, whisk together eggs, oil, sugar, and extracts. Combine the flour, baking powder, and almonds and then stir the mixture into the wet ingredients until it forms a soft dough.

- Divide the dough and form three equal loaves (9" × 3"). Place equal amounts of the sesame seeds on three pieces of wax paper. Wrap the paper around each loaf so the sesame seeds coat the entire loaf. Repeat with the remaining loaves.

- Place the loaves on a parchment paper–lined baking sheet. Bake on the middle rack for 20 minutes. Take the baking

sheet out of the oven and reduce the temperature to 300°F.

- Cool the loaves for 2 minutes. Slice each loaf along its width into ¾-inch slices with a serrated knife. Lay the slices flat on the baking sheet and

- bake them for another 10 minutes. Turn off the oven, but leave the paximadia in the oven for another 30 minutes.

- Store in a sealed container for up to 6 months.

LENTEN PAXIMADIA

These paximadia are perfect for fasting during Lent because there are no eggs in this recipe.

Makes 36

- ½ cup fresh orange juice
- 1 tablespoon grated orange zest
- ¾ cup vegetable oil
- ½ cup dry white wine
- 1½ teaspoons ground cinnamon
- ¼ teaspoon ground cloves
- ¾ cup sugar
- ¼ teaspoon baking soda
- 1½ tablespoons baking powder 1 cup chopped almonds
- 3 cups all-purpose flour
- 1 cup sesame seeds

Directions

- Preheat the oven to 350°F. Add the orange juice, zest, oil, wine, cinnamon, cloves, sugar, baking soda, and baking powder to a food processor and process until the ingredients are well incorporated. In a large bowl, stir together the almonds and flour. Pour the orange juice mixture into the flour mixture and, using a wooden spoon, combine until it forms a soft dough.

- Divide the dough and form three equal loaves (9" × 3"). Place equal amounts of sesame seeds on three pieces of wax paper. Wrap the paper around each loaf so the sesame seeds coat the entire loaf. Repeat with the remaining loaves.

- Place the loaves on a parchment paper–lined baking sheet. Bake on the middle rack for 20 minutes. Take the baking sheet out of the oven and reduce the oven to 300°F.

- Cool the loaves for 2 minutes. Slice each loaf along its width into 3⁄4-inch slices with a serrated knife. Lay the slices flat on the baking sheet, and bake them for another 10 minutes. Turn off the oven, but leave the paximadia in the oven for another 30 minutes.

- Store them in a sealed container for up to 6 months.

PAXIMADIA WITH FIGS, STAR ANISE, AND WALNUTS

Star anise is a spice that is similar to anise, but it has a more floral scent and taste.

Serves 36

- 1 cup extra-virgin olive oil
- 2 teaspoons vanilla extract
- 4 tablespoons ground star anise
- 1 ounce ouzo
- 1 cup sugar
- 3 large eggs
- 4 cups all-purpose flour
- 1 tablespoon baking powder
- 1 cup chopped dry figs
- 1 cup chopped walnuts
- 2 tablespoons petimezi (grape molasses) diluted in 2 tablespoons warm water 1 cup sesame seeds

Directions

- In a large bowl, whisk together oil, vanilla, star anise, ouzo, sugar, and eggs. In another bowl, combine the flour, baking powder, figs, and walnuts. Add the dry ingredients to the wet ingredients. Use a wooden spoon to combine the mixture until you form a soft dough.

- Divide the dough and form three equal loaves (9" × 3"). Brush the tops of the loaves with the petimezi mixture. Place equal amounts of sesame seeds on three pieces of wax paper. Wrap a sheet of paper around each loaf so the sesame seeds coat the entire loaf. Repeat with the remaining loaves.

- Place the loaves on a parchment paper–lined baking sheet. Bake them on the middle rack for 20 minutes. Take the baking sheet out of the oven and reduce the oven to 300°F.

- Cool the loaves for 2 minutes. Slice each loaf along its width into 3⁄4-inch slices with a serrated knife. Lay the slices flat on the baking sheet and bake for another 10 minutes. Turn off the oven, but leave the paximadia in the oven for another 30 minutes.

- Store in a sealed container for up to 6 months.

BOUGATSA WITH CUSTARD FILLING

Serves 12

- 2 cups melted unsalted butter, divided
- 3⁄4 cup fine semolina flour
- 1⁄2 cup granulated sugar
- 1 teaspoon vanilla extract
- 23⁄4 cups whole milk
- 24 sheets phyllo (1 package)
- 1⁄2 cup confectioners' sugar
- 2 teaspoons ground cinnamon

Directions

- In a deep, medium pot over medium heat, add 1⁄4 cup butter, semolina, sugar, and vanilla. Stir and cook for 2 minutes or until the butter is absorbed and the semolina is golden but not browned.
- Whisk in milk in a slow, steady stream until all the liquid is absorbed. Stir and cook for 3–4 minutes or until the custard has the texture of loose cream. Transfer the custard to a bowl and allow it to cool completely.
- Preheat oven to 350°F. Take phyllo sheets out of the box and lay them flat. Cover with a lightly damp kitchen towel to keep them from drying out. You will work with one sheet at a time. Keep the remaining sheets covered. Take one phyllo sheet and lay it on a clean work surface; brush the phyllo with melted butter and cover it with another phyllo sheet.
- Brush the top of the second phyllo sheet with butter as well.
- Place 3 tablespoons of custard in the center bottom third of the buttered phyllo sheets (about 2 inches from the edge). Fold the bottom 2 inches over the custard, and then fold the sides in toward the custard. Fold the phyllo up to form a package. Repeat with the remaining phyllo and custard.
- Bake the phyllo packages on a baking sheet for 15–20 minutes or until golden. Allow them to cool. Dust them with confectioners' sugar and cinnamon before serving.

FIG, APRICOT, AND ALMOND GRANOLA

Serves 16

- Nonstick vegetable oil spray
- 1⁄3 cup vegetable oil
- 1⁄3 cup honey
- 2 tablespoons white sugar
- 1 teaspoon vanilla extract
- 4 cups old-fashioned oats
- 11⁄4 cups sliced almonds
- 1⁄2 cup chopped dried apricots
- 1⁄2 cup chopped dried figs
- 1⁄2 cup (packed) brown sugar
- 1⁄2 teaspoon salt
- 1⁄2 teaspoon ground cardamom

Directions

- Preheat the oven to 300°F. Lightly spray two large baking sheets with nonstick spray.
- In a small pot over medium heat, add oil, honey, sugar, and vanilla. Cook for 5 minutes or until the sugar is dissolved. Remove the pot from the heat and let it cool for 2 minutes.
- In a large bowl, combine oats, almonds, apricots, figs, brown sugar, salt, and cardamom. Mix with your hands to combine.
- Pour the hot liquid over the dry ingredients. Using your hands (if it is too hot, use a wooden spoon), toss the ingredients together to make sure everything is well coated. Spread the granola evenly over two baking sheets. Bake for 30 minutes (stirring every 10 minutes).
- Let the granola cool completely on the baking sheets. This will allow the granola to harden before breaking it up into pieces. Store in an airtight container for up to 3 weeks.

GREEK YOGURT SMOOTHIE

Serves 4

- 2 cups Homemade Greek Yogurt (see recipe in this chapter) 2 cups orange or apple juice
- 2 large ripe bananas, peeled and chopped
- 1 cup fresh or frozen mango slices
- 1⁄2 cup fresh or frozen sliced strawberries

- 1⁄2 cup pineapple chunks
- 1⁄3 cup honey

Directions

- Put all the ingredients into the food processor.
- Process until smooth and all ingredients are well incorporated. Serve cool.

GREEK YOGURT WITH HONEY AND GRANOLA

Use store-bought granola in this recipe or try Fig, Apricot, and Almond Granola (see recipe in this chapter).

Serves 4

- 11⁄3 cups Homemade Greek Yogurt
- 1 cup granola
- 1 cup fresh berries (raspberries, blueberries, or strawberries)
- 1⁄2 cup honey

Directions

- Divide the yogurt into four small bowls and top with granola and berries.
- Drizzle honey over each bowl and serve.

GYPSY'S BREAKFAST

Serves 8

- 1 cup diced cured sausage
- 1⁄4 cup water
- 3 large potatoes, peeled and diced
- 1 large onion, peeled and sliced
- 1 large green bell pepper, stemmed, seeded, and sliced 1 large red bell pepper, stemmed, seeded, and sliced
- 1 teaspoon smoked paprika

- 3⁄4 teaspoon salt, divided
- 1⁄2 teaspoon pepper
- 1⁄2 teaspoon fresh thyme leaves
- 1 cup grated Graviera or Gruyère cheese
- 4 tablespoons extra-virgin olive oil, divided
- 8 large eggs

Directions

- In a large skillet over medium-high heat, add the sausage and water. Cook for 3 minutes or until the water evaporates and the sausage is crispy. Add the potatoes and stir to coat them in the sausage drippings. Reduce heat to medium and cook for another 5 minutes.
- Add onions, peppers, and smoked paprika. Cook for 3 more minutes. Season with 1⁄2 teaspoon salt, pepper, and thyme. Reduce heat to medium-low and cook for 10–15 minutes or until the potatoes are fork-tender. Sprinkle them with cheese and take the pan off the heat. The residual heat will melt the cheese.
- In another skillet, add 2 tablespoons oil and fry each egg to your liking (sunny-side up or over-easy). Season the eggs with the remaining salt.
- To serve, place a scoop of the vegetables onto each plate and a fried egg on top. Drizzle with remaining oil. Serve hot.

BREAKFAST BRUSCHETTA

Serves 4

- 1⁄2 loaf of Italian or French bread
- 1⁄2 cup extra-virgin olive oil
- 1⁄4 cup pesto
- 1 medium tomato
- 2 egg whites
- 2 whole eggs
- 1⁄4 cup mozzarella cheese
- 1 Roasted Red Pepper

Directions

- Slice the bread into four 3⁄4-inch lengthwise pieces. Brush one side of each with a bit of the oil; toast on grill. When that side is toasted, brush oil on the other side, flip, and toast that side.
- Place the toasted bread on a sheet pan and spread with pesto. Peel and chop the tomato; combine it with the eggs. Dice the pepper and shred the cheese.
- Heat the remaining oil in a sauté pan over medium heat; add the egg mixture and cook omelet style. Cut the omelet and place on the bread; top with cheese and pepper.

ROASTED POTATOES WITH VEGETABLES

This dish serves double duty as a treat for breakfast or as a side dish at dinner.

Serves 6

- 3 Idaho baking potatoes
- 1 sweet potato
- 3 carrots
- 1 yellow onion
- 1⁄2 pound button mushrooms

- 2 tablespoons olive oil Kosher salt, to taste
- Fresh-cracked black pepper, to taste

Directions

- Preheat the oven to 400°F.
- Large-dice the potatoes and carrots. Large-dice the onion. Trim off any discolored ends from the mushroom stems.
- In a large bowl, mix together the olive oil, potatoes, onions, carrots, and mushrooms. Place them evenly in a roasting pan, and sprinkle with salt and pepper.
- Roast the vegetables for 30–45 minutes, until tender. Serve warm.

RYE-PUMPERNICKEL STRATA WITH BLEU CHEESE

Savory breakfast is traditional in the Mediterranean. This dish is perfect to serve at brunch as well.

Serves 6

- 3 (1½-inch) slices seedless rye bread
- 3 (1½-inch) slices pumpernickel bread
- ½ teaspoon extra-virgin olive oil
- 2 whole eggs
- 6 egg whites
- ¼ cup skim milk
- ¼ cup plain nonfat yogurt 2 ounces bleu cheese Fresh-cracked black pepper, to taste

Directions

- Preheat the oven to 375°F.

- Tear the bread into large pieces. Grease a 2-quart casserole pan with the oil.
- In a large mixing bowl, beat the eggs and egg whites; add the milk, yogurt, and cheese. Place the bread pieces in the prepared casserole pan, then pour in the egg mixture. Bake for 40–50 minutes, until the mixture is set and the top is golden brown. To serve, cut into squares and season with pepper.

POLENTA

Serves 6

- 1 cup skim milk
- 2 cups favorite stock
- ½ cup cornmeal
- ¼ cup grated cheese (optional)
- Fresh-cracked black pepper, to taste

Directions

- Bring the milk and stock to a boil over medium heat in a saucepan. Slowly whisk in the cornmeal a bit at a time; stir frequently until cooked, approximately 15 minutes until mixture is the consistency of mashed potatoes. Remove from heat, add the cheese, and season with pepper.

FRUIT-STUFFED FRENCH TOAST

The rich eggy flavor of challah creates the rich profile of this dish.

Serves 6

- ½ teaspoon olive oil
- 3 small to medium loaves challah bread
- 1 pint seasonal fresh fruit

- 2 whole eggs
- 4 egg whites
- 1⁄4 cup skim milk
- 1 cup orange juice
- 1⁄4 cup nonfat plain yogurt
- 1⁄4 cup confectioners' sugar

Directions

- Preheat the oven to 375°F. Grease a baking sheet with the oil.
- Slice the bread into thick (21⁄2- to 3-inch) slices with a serrated knife at a severe angle to form long bias slices (a medium-large loaf of challah will yield three thick bias slices). Cut a slit into the bottom crust to form a pocket.
- Peel the fruit if necessary, then dice into large pieces and fill the pockets in the bread. Press the pocket closed.
- In a large mixing bowl, beat the eggs and egg whites, then add the milk. Dip the bread into the egg mixture, letting it fully absorb the mixture. Place the bread on the prepared baking sheet. Bake for 10 minutes on one side, flip, and bake 10 minutes more.
- While the bread is baking, pour the orange juice in a small saucepan; boil until reduced by half and the mixture becomes syrupy. Remove the French toast from the oven, and cut in half diagonally. Serve each with dollop of yogurt, a drizzle of juice, and a sprinkling of sugar.

PASTINA AND EGG

Pasta for breakfast? Why not—this hearty breakfast is great on a cold morning to fortify you for the day.

Serves 6

- 1 whole egg
- 2 egg whites
- 3 cups chicken broth (fat removed)
- 11⁄2 cups pastina 1 ounce fresh Parmesan cheese, grated Fresh-cracked black pepper
- 1⁄4 bunch fresh parsley, chopped

Directions

- Beat the egg and egg whites. Bring the broth to a slow boil in a medium-size saucepot, then add the pastina; stir frequently until almost al dente.
- Whisk in the eggs, stirring constantly until the eggs are completely cooked and the pasta is al dente. Remove from heat and ladle into bowls. Sprinkle in cheese, pepper, and parsley.

MEDITERRANEAN OMELETTE

Omelets in the Mediterranean are light and fluffy.

Serves 6

- 2 whole eggs
- 6 egg whites
- 1⁄4 cup plain nonfat yogurt
- 1⁄2 teaspoon extra-virgin olive oil
- 2 ounces pancetta (sliced paper-thin) or lean ham
- 3 ounces cheese (Swiss or any other), shredded

- ¼ bunch fresh parsley, chopped Fresh-cracked black pepper, to taste

Directions

- In a medium-size bowl, beat the eggs and egg whites, then whisk in the yogurt. Heat half of the oil to medium temperature in a sauté pan. Quickly sauté the pancetta, then remove and drain on paper towel.
- Heat the remaining oil to medium temperature in a large sauté pan. Pour in the egg mixture, then sprinkle in the pancetta and cheese. Stir once only. Continuously move the pan over the heat, using a spatula to push the edges inward slightly to allow the egg mixture to pour outward and solidify. When the mixture is mostly solidified, use a spatula to fold it in half.
- Cover and finish cooking on the stovetop on low heat or uncovered in a 350°F oven for approximately 5 minutes. Sprinkle with parsley and black pepper and serve.

STOVETOP-POACHED FRESH COD

A great example of a savory breakfast that provides you with protein early in the day. Great for that fresh-caught fish!

Serves 6

- 3 celery stalks
- ½ bunch fresh parsley stems
- 1½ pounds fresh cod (cut into 4-ounce portions) 1 bay leaf

- 2 cups Fish Stock
- 1 tablespoon freshly squeezed lemon juice
- Fresh black pepper, to taste
- Kosher salt, to taste

Directions

- Roughly chop the celery and parsley. Place the celery and parsley in the bottom of a sauté pan and arrange the cod pieces on top. Add the bay leaf, stock, and lemon juice, and place over medium-high heat. Cover with parchment paper or a loose-fitting lid.
- Bring to a simmer and cook covered until the fish flakes, approximately 15–20 minutes, depending on thickness of the fish. Remove from heat and season with pepper and salt; remove the bay leaf. Serve with or without poaching liquid.

SWEETENED BROWN RICE

This recipe is perfect for a cold winter day, providing a great alternative to cold cereal.

Serves 6

- 1½ cups soy milk 1½ cups water
- 1 cup brown rice
- 1 tablespoon honey
- ¼ teaspoon nutmeg Fresh fruit (optional)

Directions

- Place all the ingredients except the fresh fruit in a medium-size saucepan; bring the mixture to a slow simmer and cover with a tight-fitting lid. Simmer for 45– 60 minutes, until the rice is tender and done.

Serve in bowls, topped with your favorite fresh fruit, if desired.

CREAMY SWEET RISOTTO

This sweet version of the classic risotto can also be used for a dessert.

Serves 6

- 1 teaspoon clarified butter
- 1 teaspoon olive oil
- 1 cup Arborio rice
- 1/4 cup white grape juice 2 cups skim milk
- 1/3 cup shredded coconut
- 1/2 cup raisins or dried currants
- 3 teaspoons honey

Directions

- Heat a large sauté pan over medium heat, then add the butter and oil. Using a wooden spoon, stir in the rice. Add the juice, stirring until completely incorporated. Add the skim milk 1/4 cup at a time, stirring constantly. Make certain that each 1/4 cup is fully incorporated before adding the next.
- When the rice is completely cooked, add the coconut. Serve in bowls or on plates, sprinkled with raisins and drizzled with honey.

EGGS IN CRUSTY ITALIAN BREAD

Using crusty Italian bread is so much better than the more familiar version with empty-calorie white bread.

Serves 6

- 6 (2-inch) slices Italian bread
- 1 teaspoon virgin olive oil
- 2 red peppers, thinly sliced
- 1/2 shallot, minced 6 eggs
- Fresh-cracked black pepper, to taste
- Kosher salt, to taste

Directions

- Cut out large circles from the center of the bread slices; discard the center pieces and set the hollowed-out bread slices aside. Heat half of the oil over medium heat in a sauté pan. Sauté the peppers and shallots until tender. Remove from heat and drain on paper towel; keep warm.
- Heat the remaining oil over medium-high heat in a large sauté pan. Place the bread slices in the pan. Crack 1 egg into the hollowed-out center of each bread slice. When the eggs solidify, flip them together with the bread (being careful to keep the egg in place), and cook to desired doneness.
- To serve, top with pepper-shallot mixture, and add pepper and salt.

FRESH TUNA WITH SWEET LEMON LEEK SALSA

Serves 6

Tuna

- 1 1/2 pounds fresh tuna steaks (cut into 4-ounce portions)
- 1/4–1/2 teaspoon extra-virgin olive oil Fresh-cracked black pepper, to taste
- Kosher salt, to taste

Salsa

- 1 teaspoon extra-virgin olive oil
- 3 fresh leeks (light green and white parts only), thinly sliced
- 1 tablespoon fresh lemon juice
- 1 tablespoon honey

Directions

- Preheat grill to medium-high temperature.
- Brush each portion of the tuna with the oil and drain on a rack. Season the tuna with pepper and salt, then place the tuna on the grill; cook for 3 minutes. Shift the tuna steaks on the grill to form an X grill pattern; cook 3 more minutes.
- Turn the steaks over and grill 3 more minutes, then change position again to create an X grill pattern. Cook to desired doneness.
- **For the salsa:** Heat the oil in a medium-size sauté pan over medium heat, then add the leeks. When the leeks are wilted, add the lemon juice and honey. Plate each tuna portion with a spoonful of salsa.

YOGURT CHEESE AND FRUIT

Serves 6

- 3 cups plain nonfat yogurt
- 1 teaspoon fresh lemon juice
- 1/2 cup orange juice
- 1/2 cup water
- 1 fresh Golden Delicious apple
- 1 fresh pear
- 1/4 cup honey

- 1/4 cup dried cranberries or raisins

Directions

- Prepare the yogurt cheese the day before by lining a colander or strainer with cheesecloth. Spoon the yogurt into the cheesecloth and place the strainer over a pot or bowl to catch the whey; refrigerate for at least 8 hours before serving.
- In a large mixing bowl, mix together the juices and water. Cut the apple and pear into wedges, and place the wedges in the juice mixture; let sit for at least 5 minutes. Strain off the liquid.
- When the yogurt is firm, remove from refrigerator, slice, and place on plates. Arrange the fruit wedges around the yogurt. Drizzle with honey and sprinkle with cranberries just before serving.

PANCETTA ON BAGUETTE

This Mediterranean version of "bacon and cheese" is incredibly delicious!

Serves 6

- 1 loaf baguette
- 1/2–1 teaspoon extra-virgin olive oil
- 6 ounces pancetta (ham, prosciutto, or Canadian bacon can be substituted)
- 1/4 cantaloupe, medium-diced
- 1/4 honeydew melon, medium-diced 3 ounces goat cheese
- Fresh-cracked black pepper, to taste

Directions

- Preheat the broiler on medium-high heat.

- Slice the baguette on the bias and place on baking sheet. Brush each slice with oil, then toast lightly on each side.
- Slice the pancetta paper-thin and into thin strips, then place on top of each baguette slice; place under broiler. Cook quickly, paying close attention so as not to burn (approximately 1 minute).
- While the baguette cooks, mix the cantaloupe and melon in a small bowl. When baguettes are done, remove them from the oven and place on a plate. To serve, sprinkle with cheese and black pepper. Garnish with a spoonful of melon mix.

VEGETABLE PITA WITH FETA CHEESE

Let your imagination go wild with seasonal veggies. This simple-to-prepare pita delight is delicious, and good for you, too.

Serves 6

- 1 eggplant, sliced into 1/2-inch pieces, lengthwise 1 zucchini, sliced into 1/2-inch pieces, lengthwise 1 yellow squash, sliced
- 1 red onion, cut into 1/3-inch rings
- 1 teaspoon virgin olive oil Fresh-cracked black pepper
- 6 whole-wheat pita bread
- 3 ounces feta cheese

Directions

- Preheat the oven to 375°F.
- Brush the sliced vegetables with oil and place on a racked baking sheet. Sprinkle

with black pepper. Roast until tender. (The vegetables can be prepared the night before, refrigerated, then reheated or brought to room temperature before roasting.)
- Slice a 3-inch opening in the pitas to gain access to the pockets. Toast the pitas if desired. Fill the pitas with the cooked vegetables. Add cheese to each and serve.

ISRAELI COUSCOUS WITH DRIED-FRUIT CHUTNEY

Serves 6

- Chutney
- 1/4 cup medium-diced dried dates
- 1/4 cup medium-diced dried figs
- 1/4 cup medium-diced dried currants
- 1/4 cup slivered almonds Couscous
- 2 1/4 cups fresh orange juice
- 2 1/4 cups water
- 4 1/2 cups couscous
- 1 teaspoon grated orange rind
- 2 tablespoons nonfat plain yogurt

Directions

- Mix together all the chutney ingredients; set aside.
- Bring the orange juice and water to a boil in a medium-size pot. Stir in the couscous, then add the orange rind. Remove from heat immediately, cover, and let stand for 5 minutes. Fluff the mixture with a fork.
- Serve in bowls with a spoonful of chutney and a dollop of yogurt.

ALMOND MASCARPONE DUMPLINGS

Serves 6

- 1 cup whole-wheat flour
- 1 cup all-purpose unbleached flour
- 1⁄4 cup ground almonds 4 egg whites
- 3 ounces mascarpone cheese
- 1 teaspoon extra-virgin olive oil
- 2 teaspoons apple juice
- 1 tablespoon butter
- 1⁄4 cup honey

Directions

- Sift together both types of flour in a large bowl. Mix in the almonds. In a separate bowl, cream together the egg whites, cheese, oil, and juice on medium speed with an electric mixer.
- Combine the flour and egg white mixture with a dough hook on medium speed or by hand until a dough forms.
- Boil 1 gallon water in a medium-size saucepot. Take a spoonful of the dough and use a second spoon to push it into the boiling water. Cook until the dumpling floats to the top, about 5–10 minutes. You can cook several dumplings at once, just take care not to crowd the pot. Remove with a slotted spoon and drain on paper towels.
- Heat a medium-size sauté pan over medium-high heat. Add the butter, then place the dumplings in the pan and cook until light brown. Place on serving plates and drizzle with honey.

MULTIGRAIN TOAST WITH GRILLED VEGETABLES

Serves 6

- 1⁄2 eggplant
- 1⁄2 zucchini
- 1⁄2 yellow squash
- 1⁄2 red pepper
- 1⁄2 yellow pepper
- 1⁄2 green pepper
- 1 teaspoon extra-virgin olive oil
- 6 multigrain bread slices
- 3 ounces goat cheese
- 1⁄4 bunch fresh marjoram Fresh-cracked black pepper, to taste

Directions

- Slice the eggplant, zucchini, and squash in 3-inch lengths, 1⁄4- to 1⁄2-inch thick, and cut the peppers in half. Preheat a grill to medium heat. Brush the vegetables with the oil and grill all until fork-tender. Cut all the vegetables into large dice. (Vegetables can be prepared the night before; refrigerate and reheat or bring to room temperature before serving.)
- Grill the bread until lightly toasted, then remove from heat and top with vegetables. Sprinkle with cheese, chopped marjoram, and black pepper.

Energizing Breakfast Protein Bars

Total time: 45 minutes

Prep time: 10 minutes

Cook time: 35 minutes

Yield: 6 servings

Ingredients

- ¼ cup pecans, chopped
- 2 tbsp. pistachios, chopped
- ¼ cup flaxseeds, ground
- 1 ¼ cup spelt flakes
- ½ cup dried cherries
- 1 pinch sea salt
- ½ cup honey
- 2 tbsp. extra virgin olive oil
- ¼ cup peanut butter, natural
- ½ tsp. vanilla extract

Directions

- Start by preheating your oven to 325°F, then brush your baking tray with oil.
- Line the baking tray with parchment paper all round and brush it with oil.
- Combine the pecans, pistachios, flaxseeds, spelt, cherries, and salt in a mixing bowl and set aside.
- Place a saucepan over medium heat and pour in the honey, oil, peanut butter, and vanilla extract and cook, stirring, until the mixture melts.
- Add this mixture to the bowl of dry ingredients and mix well.
- Pour the mixture into the prepared baking tray and smooth the top.
- Bake until it turns golden brown and the sides pull out from the edges of the pan.
- Transfer the baked bar from the tray and cut it into smaller sizes on a cutting board.

- After cooling, store in an airtight container lined with parchment paper.
- The bars can last up to one week.

Fruity Nutty Muesli

Total time: 1 hour 15 minutes

Prep time 15 minutes

Cook time 1 hour

Yield: 2 servings

Ingredients

- ⅓ cup almonds, chopped
- ¾ cup oats, toasted
- ½ cup low-fat milk
- ½ cup low-fat Greek yogurt
- ½ green apple, diced
- 2 tbsp. raw honey

Directions

- Preheat oven to 350°F. Place the almonds on a baking sheet and bake until they turn golden brown, about 10 minutes.
- After cooling, mix with the toasted oats, milk and yogurt in a bowl and cover.
- Refrigerate this mixture for an hour until the oats are soft.
- Divide the muesli between two bowls, add the apple and drizzle the honey.

Egg Veggie Scramble

Total time: 30 minutes

Prep time 15 minutes

Cook time 15 minutes

Yield: 2 servings

Ingredients

- 2 tsp. extra virgin olive oil, divided

- 1 medium orange bell pepper, diced
- ½ cup frozen corn kernels
- 1 scallion, thinly sliced
- ¼ tsp. cumin, freshly ground
- ¼ tsp. allspice, plus a pinch
- 2 eggs
- 2 egg whites
- Pinch of cinnamon
- ⅓ cup white cheddar, shredded
- 1 medium avocado, diced
- ½ cup fresh salsa
- 2 whole-wheat flour tortillas, warmed

Directions

- Heat a teaspoon of olive oil in a nonstick pan over medium heat.
- Add bell pepper, tossing and turning for 5 minutes until soft; add the corn, scallion, cumin, and allspice and cook for a further 3 minutes until the scallion wilts.
- Pour this out onto a plate and cover it with foil. Wipe the pan clean with a paper towel and set it aside.
- Place the eggs and egg whites in a bowl and whisk them together with 2 teaspoons of water, a pinch of allspice and a pinch of cinnamon.
- Heat the remaining olive oil in the pan over medium heat and add the egg mixture.
- Cook until the bottom sets, about 30 seconds, then stir gently.
- Continue stirring for about 2 minutes, then add the shredded cheese and vegetables that you had wrapped in foil.

Serve with avocado, salsa and the tortillas.

MEDITERRANEAN LUNCH RECIPE

Quinoa Salad with Watermelon and Feta

Serves: 4

Ingredients

- 1 cup Simple Truth Organic™ Quinoa
- 3 tablespoons apple cider vinegar
- 2 tablespoons lemon juice
- ½ Vidalia onion, finely chopped
- ½ cup Simple Truth Organic™ Unfiltered Extra Virgin Olive Oil
- Coarse salt, to taste
- Freshly ground pepper, to taste
- ¾ cup crumbled feta cheese
- ½ seedless watermelon, (about 1½ cups) diced
- 3 tablespoons Italian parsley, minced

Directions

- Cook quinoa according to package directions. Rinse with cold water and drain.
- To make dressing: in a small bowl or jar, combine vinegar, lemon juice and onion. Mix well and add in olive oil and whisk well to emulsify dressing. Season with salt and pepper to taste.
- In a medium bowl, combine the cooked quinoa with feta, watermelon, parsley and dressing. Add salt and pepper to

taste. Serve chilled or at room temperature.

Mediterranean Orzo

Serves: 8

Ingredients

- 14 ounces orzo pasta
- 1 tablespoon Simple Extra Virgin Olive Oil
- 1 jar (8.5 oz.) sun-dried tomatoes in oil, julienne cut
- 8 green onions, chopped
- 4 ounces feta cheese
- 1/4 cup provolone cheese, shredded
- 1 jar (16 oz.) Italian dressing

Directions

- Cook pasta in a large saucepan of boiling water with 1 tablespoon olive oil. Cook until done but still firm to bite. Drain and allow to cool.
- In a large bowl, combine pasta, sun-dried tomatoes, green onions, feta cheese and provolone. Pour dressing over top. Stir to combine.

Meyer Lemon Quinoa Skillet

Ingredients

- 2 teaspoons olive oil
- 1/2 cup onion, chopped
- 1 teaspoon minced garlic
- 1 can (15.5 oz.) cannellini beans, drained and rinsed
- 1 can (14 oz.) quartered artichoke hearts, drained and roughly chopped
- 2 packages (10 oz.) Simple Truth Organic White Quinoa with Olive Oil & Sea Salt
- 1/4 cup water
- 2 Meyer lemons, zested and juiced
- 1/2 teaspoon salt
- 1/4 teaspoon ground black pepper
- 2 tablespoons flat leaf parsley, chopped
- 4 ounces crumbled feta cheese

Directions

- In medium non-stick skillet over medium heat, heat oil. Cook onion and garlic 2 to 3 minutes, until translucent.
- Stir in beans, artichokes, quinoa and water. Cook 4 to 6 minutes until hot.
- Stir in lemon juice, salt, pepper and parsley. Adjust seasoning to taste.
- Serve topped with feta cheese and lemon zest.

Creamy Corn, Squash and Cilantro

Serves: 8

Ingredients

- 4 cloves garlic, minced and divided
- 1/4 cup cilantro, minced
- 1/2 cup mayonnaise
- 2 tablespoons sour cream
- 1/4 teaspoon salt
- 1 bag (10 oz.) Simple Truth Organic™ Whole Kernel Cut Corn
- 3 tablespoons Olive oil
- 1 zucchini, washed and chopped
- 1 yellow squash, washed and chopped

- 1/2 cup queso fresco, crumbled

Directions

- Heat grill to 250°F.
- To make aioli, mix 2 garlic cloves, mayonnaise, sour cream and salt in a small bowl.
- Cook corn in microwave as directed on the package.
- Heat oil in cast iron skillet and place on the grill. Add 2 minced garlic cloves and cook, uncovered, for 30 seconds. Add zucchini and yellow squash and cook for 3-5 minutes, turning occasionally, until vegetables are crisp-tender. Add corn and cook until vegetables are cooked through.
- Serve vegetables with aioli and queso fresco on the side.

Mediterranean Turkey and Rice Skillet

Serves: 5

Ingredients

- 1 tablespoon olive oil
- 1 pound ground turkey
- 1 small onion, chopped
- 2 teaspoons minced garlic
- 1 teaspoon salt
- 1/2 teaspoon ground black pepper
- 1/2 teaspoon dried oregano
- 1/2 cup Private Selection Sun-Dried Tomatoes, drained and roughly chopped
- 1 cup long grain white rice
- 2 cups chicken broth
- 5 ounces baby spinach

- 1 lemon, zested and juiced
- 1/2 cup feta cheese crumbles

Directions

- In large skillet over medium-high heat, heat oil. Cook ground turkey, onion, garlic, salt, pepper and oregano until meat is browned and onion is translucent.
- Mix in sun-dried tomatoes, rice and chicken broth. Bring to boil. Cover and reduce heat to low. Cook 15 minutes, until rice is tender.
- Stir in spinach, lemon juice and zest. Continue cooking until spinach is wilted.
- Serve topped with feta cheese.

Mediterranean Quinoa Stuffed Peppers

Ingredients

- 2 large red bell peppers
- 1 cup cooked quinoa
- 1 cup low sodium cooked chickpeas
- 1 cup cherry tomatoes, quartered
- 2 tablespoons pine nuts
- 2 tablespoons sliced black olives
- 1 clove garlic
- 1 teaspoon red wine vinegar
- 1 teaspoon dried oregano
- Chopped parsley, for serving (optional)

Preparation

- Heat oven to 350F.
- Cut bell peppers vertically down the center in half and remove stems and seeds. Place peppers on a baking sheet

lined with parchment or a silicone baking mat.

- In a mixing bowl, combine remaining ingredients. Scoop mixture into pepper halves.
- Bake for 20 to 25 minutes, or until peppers are soft but still hold their shape. Remove from oven and sprinkle with parsley before serving (optional).

Japanese Onigiri Rice Triangles Recipe

Ingredients

- 1½ cups uncooked short grain white rice
- 1 2/3 cups water
- ½ teaspoon salt
- ½ ounce dried sliced seaweed, finely chopped (2 tablespoons)
- 1 tablespoon sesame seeds
- 4 ounces cooked, smoked, or canned salmon
- 1 sheet nori

Preparation

- Measure the rice in a medium saucepan. Rinse, stir, and drain it several times. Cover it with plenty of water and allow it to soak for about 40 minutes or until the rice is an opaque white color. Thoroughly drain the rice in a mesh strainer.
- Return the drained rice to the saucepan. Add water and salt; cover the pot. Bring it to a boil over high heat, then reduce heat to maintain a simmer. Cook the rice for 20 minutes, then remove it from the heat. Leave the pot covered and allow the rice

to steam for another 10 minutes to finish the cooking process.

- Sprinkle in the seaweed and sesame seeds. Stir to combine.
- When the rice mixture is cool enough to handle, moisten both hands. Spread about ½ cup of the rice out on the palm of one hand. Place 1 tablespoon of salmon in the center, and form the rice mixture into a ball around it. Press firmly to stick the rice together. Form it into the traditional triangle shape, flat on both sides, with rounded corners.
- Using scissors, cut the sheet of nori into strips, 1 x 2 ½-inches each; wrap a strip of nori around one edge of the triangle. Cover or wrap tightly until serving.

Maple Pumpkin Pie Buckwheat Groats

Ingredients

- ½ cup raw buckwheat groats
- 2/3 cup unsweetened almond milk beverage
- ½ teaspoon pumpkin pie spice
- 1/8 teaspoon salt
- ½ teaspoon vanilla extract
- 4 teaspoons 100% pure maple syrup

Preparation

- Place groats in a bowl and cover them with water. Place groats in the refrigerator to soak overnight. The next day, drain the groats. It is normal for buckwheat to be somewhat mucilaginous, so groats will be slippery. Rinse well and drain again.

- To a 2-quart saucepan, add the groats, almond milk, pumpkin pie spice, and salt, and whisk to dissolve the spices. Cover and bring to a boil, then reduce heat to a low simmer and cook for 4 minutes. Remove cover and turn heat up to maintain a simmer and cook for an additional 2 minutes, stirring occasionally.
- Remove from the heat and stir in vanilla and maple syrup.

Chicken, Broccoli, and Rice Casserole Recipe

Ingredients

- 12 ounces boneless, skinless chicken breast
- 1/4 teaspoon sea salt
- 3/4 teaspoon freshly cracked black pepper, divided
- 2 tablespoons olive oil, divided
- 1/2 medium yellow onion, diced
- 2 cloves garlic, minced
- 3 cups frozen broccoli florets
- 1 tablespoon whole wheat flour or all-purpose flour
- 1 1/2 cups skim milk
- 3/4 cups sharp cheddar cheese, freshly grated, divided
- 2 cups cooked whole grain wild rice blend
- Cooking spray
- 1/4 cup whole wheat panko breadcrumbs

Preparation

- Heat oven to 350F. Cut chicken into 1/2-inch cubes. Season with salt and 1/4 teaspoon pepper.
- In a large skillet, heat 1/2 tablespoon of the oil over medium heat. Add chicken and cook, stirring, until chicken is cooked through. Remove chicken to a large bowl.
- In the same skillet, heat another 1/2 tablespoon of oil. Add garlic, onion, and broccoli. Cook, stirring until onion is soft and broccoli is bright green. Pour into bowl with chicken.
- Turn heat to low and add the remaining tablespoon of oil to the skillet. Sprinkle flour over oil and whisk to make a paste. Slowly add milk, whisking to combine. Stir in cheese and remaining 1/2 teaspoon of black pepper. Remove from heat.
- Add rice to chicken and broccoli in the large bowl. Stir to combine. Gently stir in cheese sauce.
- Spray a 9x9-inch baking dish with cooking spray. Spread rice mixture into baking dish. Sprinkle with remaining 1/4 cup of cheese and breadcrumbs.
- Bake 15 to 20 minutes, or until cheese is melted and casserole is bubbly. Remove from the oven and serve hot

Baked Coconut Rice

Ingredients

- 1 tablespoon coconut oil
- 2 cups uncooked brown jasmine rice

- 1 teaspoon salt
- 13.5-ounce can coconut milk
- 2 cups water
- ½ cup slivered fresh pineapple
- ¼ cup toasted coconut flakes
- ¼ cup toasted sliced almonds

Preparation

- Preheat the oven to 375F.
- In a 4-quart ovenproof pot, melt the coconut oil over medium heat on the stovetop. Rinse and drain the rice in a mesh strainer and add it to the coconut oil. Brown the rice, stirring occasionally, for 5 minutes. Add the salt, coconut milk, and water. Bring the rice to a boil.
- Cover the pot tightly with a heavy lid or aluminum foil and place it in the oven. Bake for 35 minutes. Test it to make sure it is almost tender. If it isn't almost tender, add another quarter cup of water and return it to the oven for another 10 minutes. Allow the rice to rest, covered, for 5 more minutes to complete the cooking process. Fluff and serve the rice, garnished with slivered pineapple, coconut flakes, and sliced almonds.

Healthy Butternut Squash Grain Bowl

Ingredients

- 1 cup butternut squash cubes
- 1 teaspoon olive oil
- 1 teaspoon maple syrup
- 1/4 teaspoon cinnamon
- 1/4 teaspoon freshly cracked pepper

- Pinch salt
- 1/4 cup pecans
- 1 cup cooked wild rice
- 2 cups baby spinach or spring mix
- 1 small Honeycrisp apple
- 1/4 cup dried cranberries

Preparation

- Heat oven to 400F. Line a baking sheet with parchment or a silicone baking mat.
- Toss butternut squash with oil, syrup, cinnamon, pepper, and salt. Spread evenly on the baking sheet and roast for 25 to 30 minutes, stirring occasionally.
- Place pecans on a piece of foil or small baking sheet and toast at 400F for 5 to 10 minutes or until fragrant, watching carefully.
- Assemble bowls. Divide rice between two bowls. Add greens, squash, apples, cranberries and toasted pecans.

Low Sodium Garlic Parmesan Popcorn

Ingredients

- 2 teaspoons olive or avocado oil
- 1/4 cup popcorn kernels
- 2 cloves garlic, minced
- 2 tablespoons good quality parmesan cheese, freshly grated
- 1/4 teaspoon garlic powder

Preparation

- Heat oil in the bottom of a small saucepan over medium high heat. Add 2 or 3 kernels to the pan while heating.

- Once kernels start to pop, add remaining popcorn kernels and garlic. Cover the pan and cook, shaking the pan to keep kernels from burning.
- Once kernels have stopped popping, remove from heat and sprinkle the parmesan and garlic powder on top. Shake to coat popcorn evenly, then pour into bowls and enjoy.

Gluten-Free Coconut Granola

Ingredients

- 3 cups certified gluten-free rolled oats
- ½ cup sweetened shredded coconut
- ¼ teaspoon kosher salt
- 1/3 cup maple syrup
- 1 tablespoon canola oil
- ½ cup sliced almonds
- 1 cup dried cranberries

Preparation

- Preheat oven to 325°F.
- Line a large sheet pan with parchment paper; set aside.
- Combine gluten free oats, coconut, salt, maple syrup, and canola oil in a large bowl.
- Toss ingredients well and pour out onto a prepared baking sheet.
- Bake, stirring occasionally, until golden brown (15 to 20 minutes).
- Remove from oven to cool.
- Once cool, mix in almonds and dried cranberries.
- Enjoy right away or store in an airtight container for up to 2 weeks.

Simple Black Bean and Barley Vegetarian Burritos

Ingredients

- 1/2 cup barley, dry
- 1 tablespoon olive oil
- 1 small onion, chopped
- 1 teaspoon dry garlic
- pinch red pepper flakes
- 1/4 teaspoon cumin
- 1/4 teaspoon salt
- 3 tablespoons tomato paste
- 1 medium carrot, shredded
- 1 15-ounce can black beans
- 6 large whole wheat tortillas (9 or 10 inches across)
- avocado, salsa, shredded cheddar, or sour cream, for garnish and dipping, optional

Preparation

- Prepare barley according to package instructions.
- While barley is cooking, heat up olive oil in a medium-sized pan over medium heat. Add onion, garlic, pepper flakes, cumin, salt, tomato paste, carrot, and black beans. Stir together and let heat for about 5 minutes. Remove from heat and mash the mixture slightly with a fork.
- Once barley is ready, place each tortilla on a separate plate. Divide the barley and black bean mixture into six parts and arrange them towards the middle of each tortilla.

Pecan Brown Butter Oat Triangles Recipe

Ingredients

- ½ cup pecan halves
- ½ cup butter
- ¼ cup light corn syrup
- ½ cup packed light brown sugar
- 1/8 teaspoon salt
- 1 teaspoon vanilla extract
- 2 ½ cups rolled oats

Preparation

- Preheat the oven to 350F. Line an 8- by an 8-inch baking dish with parchment (no greasing needed), or line with generously greased foil and set aside.
- Place pecans on a baking sheet and toast in the middle of the oven until they are 1 or 2 shades darker, 7 to 9 minutes, stirring once after 4 minutes. Watch carefully to prevent burning. Remove from the oven, pour into a small bowl and place nuts in the freezer to cool until they can be handled safely. Once they are cool, coarsely chop the pecans.
- In a 2-quart saucepan over medium-high heat, melt the butter while swirling the pan periodically. Adjust the heat to maintain gentle bubbling until foam turns a very light golden color and the liquid butter underneath begins to brown, 3 to 4 minutes. Continue to cook and swirl the pan until the liquid butter under the foam turns copper-colored, 2 to 3 minutes more. Remove the pan from the heat and stir in the corn syrup until dissolved. Stir in the brown sugar and salt and return to heat. Boil for 1 minute. Remove pan from heat again and stir in vanilla.
- Add oats and pecans to the saucepan and stir to coat. Pour the mixture into the prepared baking dish and spread evenly. Place a small piece of parchment paper or oiled foil on top of oats and press down firmly with your hand to flatten, paying attention to sides and corners. Use care: the mixture is still quite hot. Bake in the middle of the oven until the edges turn light golden brown, 13 to 15 minutes.
- Remove from the oven and place on a cooling rack for 15 minutes. Remove the whole bar from the pan by lifting the edges of the parchment paper and place it on a cutting board. While still warm, use a large chef's knife to cut the bar into 16 squares. Cut each square diagonally into 2 triangles (1 3/4 x 1 3/4 x 2 1/2-inch) to make 32 pieces. Cool completely, then store in an airtight container.

Golden Pilaf

Yield: 6 servings

- 2 teaspoons olive oil
- 1 medium onion, chopped
- 1/4 cup golden raisins
- 1 cup long-grain rice
- 1/2 teaspoon turmeric
- 1/8 teaspoon cinnamon
- 1/8 teaspoon cardamom

- 2 cups low-sodium chicken or vegetable stock
- 1/4 cup pistachios, chopped
- 1/4 cup parsley, chopped

Directions

- In a 2-quart saucepan, heat the olive oil over medium-high heat. Add the onions and raisins and sauté for 3 minutes.
- Stir in the rice, turmeric, cinnamon, and cardamom and sauté for 1 minute. Add the stock, bring the mixture to a boil, and cover.
- Reduce the heat to a simmer for 15 to 18 minutes or until the liquid is fully absorbed.
- Meanwhile, toast the pistachios in small nonstick skillet for 1 minute or until fragrant. Add the pistachios and parsley to the cooked rice and serve.

Per serving: Calories 205 (From Fat 43); Fat 5g (Saturated 1g); Cholesterol 0mg; Sodium 48mg; Carbohydrate 36g (Dietary Fiber 2g); Protein 6g.

Wild Rice Pilaf

- 2 cups wild rice, cooked
- 2 cups orzo, cooked
- 2 cups baby spinach leaves, chopped
- 1/4 cup kalamata olives, pitted
- 1/4 cup fresh dill, chopped
- 1/4 cup fresh parsley, chopped
- 1/4 cup olive oil
- Juice of 1 lemon
- 1 cup grape tomatoes, halved lengthwise
- Salt and pepper to taste
- 2 ounces feta cheese, crumbled

Directions

- In a large bowl, combine the rice, orzo, spinach, olives, dill, and olive oil. Toss to coat.
- Add the lemon juice and gently stir in the tomatoes and parsley. Season with salt and pepper to taste. Top with the cheese and serve.

Moroccan Couscous

- 1-1/2 cups vegetable stock
- Zest and juice of 1 orange
- 1/3 cup chopped dates
- 1/3 cup chopped dried apricots
- 1/3 cup golden raisins
- 1/4 teaspoon ground cinnamon
- 1/2 teaspoon ground cumin
- 1/4 teaspoon coriander
- 1/2 teaspoon ground ginger
- 1/2 teaspoon turmeric
- 2 cups dry plain or whole-wheat couscous
- 1 tablespoon butter
- 1/2 cup slivered almonds, toasted
- 1/4 cup mint, chopped
- Salt to taste

Directions

- In a medium saucepan, bring the stock to a boil. Add the orange juice and zest, dates, apricots, raisins, spices, and couscous.
- Cover and remove the pan from the heat.
- Allow the couscous to absorb the liquid, about 15 minutes. If your couscous is too dry, add a bit of water, cover, and wait 5

minutes; repeat until the couscous is the desired consistency.

- Uncover, add the butter, and mix well. Stir in the almonds and mint and season with salt to taste before serving.

Couscous with Tomatoes and Cucumbers

- 2 cups water
- 1 cup whole-wheat couscous
- 1/2 teaspoon coriander
- 2 Roma or plum tomatoes, chopped
- 1 small cucumber, seeded and chopped
- 1/2 medium red onion, chopped
- One 14.5-ounce can chickpeas, drained and rinsed
- 1/2 cup fresh mint, chopped
- 1/3 cup lemon juice
- 1 tablespoon olive oil
- Salt and pepper to taste

Directions

- In a medium saucepan, bring the water to a boil.
- Stir in the couscous and coriander, cover, and remove from the heat. Allow the couscous to absorb the liquid completely, about 15 minutes.
- Combine the cooked couscous with the tomatoes, cucumber, onions, chickpeas, and mint in a large bowl.
- Whisk together the lemon juice and olive oil, pour the mixture over the couscous salad, and stir well.
- Cover and refrigerate for at least 2 hours. Serve.

Charcuterie Bistro Lunch Box

Ingredients

- 1 slice prosciutto
- 1 mozzarella stick, halved
- 2 breadsticks, halved
- 2 dates
- ½ cup grapes
- 2 large radishes, halved or 4 slices English cucumber (1/4-inch)

Directions

- Cut prosciutto in half lengthwise, then wrap a slice around each portion of cheese. Arrange the wrapped cheese, breadsticks, dates, grapes and radishes (or cucumber) in a 4-cup divided sealable container. Keep refrigerated until ready to eat.

Mediterranean Chicken Quinoa Bowl

Ingredients

- 1 pound boneless, skinless chicken breasts, trimmed
- ¼ teaspoon salt
- ¼ teaspoon ground pepper
- 1 7-ounce jar roasted red peppers, rinsed
- ¼ cup slivered almonds
- 4 tablespoons extra-virgin olive oil, divided
- 1 small clove garlic, crushed
- 1 teaspoon paprika
- ½ teaspoon ground cumin

- ¼ teaspoon crushed red pepper (Optional)
- 2 cups cooked quinoa
- ¼ cup pitted Kalamata olives, chopped
- ¼ cup finely chopped red onion
- 1 cup diced cucumber
- ¼ cup crumbled feta cheese
- 2 tablespoons finely chopped fresh parsley

Directions

- Position a rack in upper third of oven; preheat broiler to high. Line a rimmed baking sheet with foil.
- Sprinkle chicken with salt and pepper and place on the prepared baking sheet. Broil, turning once, until an instant-read thermometer inserted in the thickest part reads 165 degrees F, 14 to 18 minutes. Transfer the chicken to a clean cutting board and slice or shred.
- Meanwhile, place peppers, almonds, 2 tablespoons oil, garlic, paprika, cumin and crushed red pepper (if using) in a mini food processor. Puree until fairly smooth.
- Combine quinoa, olives, red onion and the remaining 2 tablespoons oil in a medium bowl.
- To serve, divide the quinoa mixture among 4 bowls and top with equal amounts of cucumber, the chicken and the red pepper sauce. Sprinkle with feta and parsley.

Mediterranean Lettuce Wraps

Ingredients

- ¼ cup tahini
- ¼ cup extra-virgin olive oil
- 1 teaspoon lemon zest
- ¼ cup lemon juice (from 2 lemons)
- 1 ½ teaspoons pure maple syrup
- ¾ teaspoon kosher salt
- ½ teaspoon paprika
- 2 (15 ounce) cans no-salt-added chickpeas, rinsed
- ½ cup sliced jarred roasted red peppers, drained
- ½ cup thinly sliced shallots
- 12 large Bibb lettuce leaves
- ¼ cup toasted almonds, chopped
- 2 tablespoons chopped fresh parsley

Directions

- Whisk tahini, oil, lemon zest, lemon juice, maple syrup, salt and paprika in a large bowl. Add chickpeas, peppers and shallots. Toss to coat.
- Divide the mixture among lettuce leaves (about 1/3 cup each). Top with almonds and parsley. Wrap the lettuce leaves around the filling and serve.

Salmon Pita Sandwich

Ingredients

- 2 tablespoons plain nonfat yogurt
- 2 teaspoons chopped fresh dill
- 2 teaspoons lemon juice
- ½ teaspoon prepared horseradish

- 3 ounces flaked drained canned sockeye salmon
- ½ 6-inch whole-wheat pita bread
- ½ cup watercress

Directions

- Combine yogurt, dill, lemon juice and horseradish in a small bowl; stir in salmon. Stuff the pita half with the salmon salad and watercress.

Hummus & Greek Salad

Ingredients

- 2 cups arugula
- ⅓ cup cherry tomatoes, halved
- ⅓ cup sliced cucumber
- 1 tablespoon chopped red onion
- 1 ½ tablespoons extra-virgin olive oil
- 2 teaspoons red-wine vinegar
- ⅛ teaspoon ground pepper
- 1 tablespoon feta cheese
- 1 4-inch whole-wheat pita
- ¼ cup hummus

Directions

- Toss arugula in a bowl with tomatoes, cucumber, onion, oil, vinegar and pepper. Top with feta. Serve with pita and hummus.

Mediterranean Wrap

Ingredients

- ½ cup water
- ⅓ cup couscous, preferably whole-wheat
- 1 cup chopped fresh parsley
- ½ cup chopped fresh mint

- ¼ cup lemon juice
- 3 tablespoons extra-virgin olive oil
- 2 teaspoons minced garlic
- ¼ teaspoon salt, divided
- ¼ teaspoon freshly ground pepper
- 1 pound chicken tenders
- 1 medium tomato, chopped
- 1 cup chopped cucumber
- 4 10-inch spinach or sun-dried tomato wraps or tortillas

Directions

- Bring water to a boil in a small saucepan. Stir in couscous and remove from the heat. Cover and let stand for 5 minutes. Fluff with a fork. Set aside.
- Meanwhile, combine parsley, mint, lemon juice, oil, garlic, 1/8 teaspoon salt and pepper in a small bowl.
- Toss chicken tenders in a medium bowl with 1 tablespoon of the parsley mixture and the remaining 1/8 teaspoon salt. Place the tenders in a large nonstick skillet and cook over medium heat until cooked though, 3 to 5 minutes per side. Transfer to a clean cutting board. Cut into bite-size pieces when cool enough to handle.
- Stir the remaining parsley mixture into the couscous along with tomato and cucumber.
- To assemble wraps, spread about 3/4 cup of the couscous mixture onto each wrap. Divide the chicken among the wraps. Roll the wraps up like a burrito,

tucking in the sides to hold the ingredients in. Serve cut in half.

Mediterranean Bento Lunch

Ingredients

- ¼ cup chickpeas, rinsed
- ¼ cup diced cucumber
- ¼ cup diced tomato
- 1 tablespoon diced olives
- 1 tablespoon crumbled feta cheese
- 1 tablespoon chopped fresh parsley
- ½ teaspoon extra-virgin olive oil
- 1 teaspoon red-wine vinegar
- 3 ounces grilled turkey breast tenderloin or chicken breast
- 1 cup grapes
- 1 whole-wheat pita bread, quartered
- 2 tablespoons hummus

Directions

- Toss chickpeas, cucumber, tomato, olives, feta, parsley, oil and vinegar together in a medium bowl. Pack in a medium-sized container.
- Place turkey (or chicken) in a medium container.
- Pack grapes and pita in small containers and hummus in a dip-size container.

Greek Chicken & Cucumber Pita Sandwiches with Yogurt Sauce

Ingredients

- 1 teaspoon lemon zest
- 2 tablespoons fresh lemon juice
- 5 teaspoons olive oil, divided
- 1 tablespoon chopped fresh oregano or 1 teaspoon dried
- 2 ¾ teaspoons minced garlic, divided
- ¼ teaspoon crushed red pepper
- 1 pound chicken tenders
- 1 English cucumber, halved, seeded and grated, plus 1/2 English cucumber, halved and sliced
- ½ teaspoon salt, divided
- ¾ cup nonfat plain Greek yogurt
- 2 teaspoons chopped fresh mint
- 2 teaspoons chopped fresh dill
- 1 teaspoon ground pepper
- 2 (6 1/2 inch) whole-wheat pita breads, halved
- 4 lettuce leaves
- ½ cup sliced red onion
- 1 cup chopped plum tomatoes

Directions

- Combine lemon zest, lemon juice, 3 tsp. oil, oregano, 2 tsp. garlic, and crushed red pepper in a large bowl. Add chicken and toss to coat. Marinate in the refrigerator for at least 1 hour or up to 4 hours.
- Meanwhile, toss grated cucumber with 1/4 tsp. salt in a fine-mesh sieve. Let drain for 15 minutes, then squeeze to release more liquid. Transfer to a medium bowl. Stir in yogurt, mint, dill, ground pepper, and the remaining 2 tsp. oil, 3/4 tsp. garlic, and 1/4 tsp. salt. Refrigerate until ready to serve.
- Preheat grill to medium-high.

- Oil the grill rack (see Tip). Grill the chicken until an instant-read thermometer inserted in the center registers 165 degrees F, 3 to 4 minutes per side.
- To serve, spread some of the sauce inside each pita half. Tuck in the chicken, lettuce, red onion, tomatoes, and sliced cucumber.

Slow-Cooker Mediterranean Chicken & Chickpea Soup

Ingredients

- 1 ½ cups dried chickpeas, soaked overnight
- 4 cups water
- 1 large yellow onion, finely chopped
- 1 (15 ounce) can no-salt-added diced tomatoes, preferably fire-roasted
- 2 tablespoons tomato paste
- 4 cloves garlic, finely chopped
- 1 bay leaf
- 4 teaspoons ground cumin
- 4 teaspoons paprika
- ¼ teaspoon cayenne pepper
- ¼ teaspoon ground pepper
- 2 pounds bone-in chicken thighs, skin removed, trimmed
- 1 (14 ounce) can artichoke hearts, drained and quartered
- ¼ cup halved pitted oil-cured olives
- ½ teaspoon salt
- ¼ cup chopped fresh parsley or cilantro

Directions

- Drain chickpeas and place in a 6-quart or larger slow cooker. Add 4 cups water, onion, tomatoes and their juice, tomato paste, garlic, bay leaf, cumin, paprika, cayenne and ground pepper; stir to combine. Add chicken.
- Cover and cook on Low for 8 hours or High for 4 hours.
- Transfer the chicken to a clean cutting board and let cool slightly. Discard bay leaf. Add artichokes, olives and salt to the slow cooker and stir to combine. Shred the chicken, discarding bones. Stir the chicken into the soup. Serve topped with parsley (or cilantro).

Prosciutto, Mozzarella & Melon Plate

Ingredients

- 1 cup cubed cantaloupe
- 6 thin slices prosciutto, cut in half
- 10 small fresh mozzarella balls
- ½ cup cherry tomato halves
- 6 (1/4 inch thick) slices whole-wheat baguette
- ½ cup unsalted hazelnuts
- 4 chocolate-dipped strawberries

Directions

- Divide items equally among 2 plates.

Tips

- Want to try making your own chocolate-covered strawberries? Try these deliciously boozy Chocolate-Covered Prosecco Strawberries.

- To make ahead: Pack ingredients in separate totable containers.

Mediterranean Pasta Salad

Ingredients

- 2 tablespoons plain hummus
- 1 tablespoon water
- 2 teaspoons extra-virgin olive oil
- ½ cup chopped red bell pepper
- ½ cup canned quartered artichoke hearts, drained and cut in half
- 1 cup lightly packed baby kale
- 4 pitted Kalamata olives, roughly chopped
- 1 (3 ounce) can no-salt-added light tuna in water, drained
- ½ cup cooked farfalle, preferably whole-wheat
- 1 tablespoon crumbled feta cheese
- 1 tablespoon toasted chopped walnuts
- 1 tablespoon Juice from 1/4 lemon

Directions

- Whisk hummus and water in a small bowl. Set aside.
- Heat oil in a medium nonstick skillet over medium-high heat. Add bell pepper; cook for 1 minute. Add artichoke hearts, kale, and olives. Gently stir in tuna, trying not to not break up large pieces; cook until the tuna is warmed, about 1 minute more. Stir in pasta. Remove from heat and toss with the hummus sauce. Top with feta and walnuts and drizzle with lemon juice, if desired.

Tips

- To make ahead: Cook pasta up to 1 day ahead and refrigerate.

Mediterranean Chickpea Quinoa Bowl

Ingredients

- 1 (7 ounce) jar roasted red peppers, rinsed
- ¼ cup slivered almonds
- 4 tablespoons extra-virgin olive oil, divided
- 1 small clove garlic, minced
- 1 teaspoon paprika
- ½ teaspoon ground cumin
- ¼ teaspoon crushed red pepper (optional)
- 2 cups cooked quinoa
- ¼ cup Kalamata olives, chopped
- ¼ cup finely chopped red onion
- 1 (15 ounce) can chickpeas, rinsed
- 1 cup diced cucumber
- ¼ cup crumbled feta cheese
- 2 tablespoons finely chopped fresh parsley

Directions

- Place peppers, almonds, 2 tablespoons oil, garlic, paprika, cumin and crushed red pepper (if using) in a mini food processor. Puree until fairly smooth.
- Combine quinoa, olives, red onion and the remaining 2 tablespoons oil in a medium bowl.
- To serve, divide the quinoa mixture among 4 bowls and top with equal

amounts of the chickpeas, cucumber and the red pepper sauce. Sprinkle with feta and parsley.

Mediterranean Lentil & Kale Salad

Ingredients

- ¼ cup red wine vinegar
- 2 tablespoons olive oil
- 1 tablespoon finely chopped dried tomatoes (not oil-packed)
- 1 clove garlic, minced
- ½ teaspoon Dijon-style mustard
- ¼ teaspoon salt
- ¼ teaspoon black pepper
- 1 5-ounce package (8 cups) fresh baby kale
- 1 9-ounce package refrigerated steamed lentils, such as Melissa
- 1 cup chopped red sweet pepper
- ¼ cup shredded Parmesan cheese (1/2 ounce)

Directions

- For vinaigrette, in a large serving bowl whisk together the red wine vinegar, olive oil, chopped dried tomatoes, garlic, mustard, salt and pepper. Add kale; toss to coat. Top with lentils and sweet pepper and sprinkle with cheese.

Ravioli & Vegetable Soup

Ingredients

- 1 tablespoon extra-virgin olive oil

- 2 cups frozen bell pepper and onion mix, thawed and diced
- 2 cloves garlic, minced
- 1/4 teaspoon crushed red pepper, or to taste (optional)
- 1 28-ounce can crushed tomatoes, preferably fire-roasted
- 1 15-ounce can vegetable broth or reduced-sodium chicken broth
- 1 ½ cups hot water
- 1 teaspoon dried basil or marjoram
- 1 6- to 9-ounce package fresh or frozen cheese (or meat) ravioli, preferably whole-wheat
- 2 cups diced zucchini, (about 2 medium)
- Freshly ground pepper to taste

Directions

- Heat oil in a large saucepan or Dutch oven over medium heat. Add pepper-onion mix, garlic and crushed red pepper (if using) and cook, stirring, for 1 minute.
- Add tomatoes, broth, water and basil (or marjoram); bring to a rolling boil over high heat. Add ravioli and cook for 3 minutes less than the package directions.
- Add zucchini; return to a boil. Cook until the zucchini is crisp-tender, about 3 minutes. Season with pepper.

Mediterranean Tuna-Spinach Salad

Ingredients

- 1 ½ tablespoons tahini
- 1 ½ tablespoons lemon juice

- 1 ½ tablespoons water
- 1 5-ounce can chunk light tuna in water, drained
- 4 Kalamata olives, pitted and chopped
- 2 tablespoons feta cheese
- 2 tablespoons parsley
- 2 cups baby spinach
- 1 medium orange, peeled or sliced

Directions

- Whisk tahini, lemon juice and water together in a bowl. Add tuna, olives, feta and parsley; stir to combine.
- Serve the tuna salad over 2 cups spinach, with the orange on the side.

Italian Pesto Chicken Salad

Ingredients

- ½ cup nonfat plain Greek yogurt
- ⅓ cup mayonnaise
- 2 tablespoons minced shallot
- 2 tablespoons pesto
- 2 teaspoons lemon juice
- ½ teaspoon salt
- ½ teaspoon ground pepper
- 3 cups shredded or chopped cooked chicken
- 1 cup packed coarsely chopped arugula
- ½ cup halved cherry tomatoes
- 3 tablespoons toasted pine nuts

Directions

- Combine yogurt, mayonnaise, shallot, pesto, lemon juice, salt and pepper in a large bowl. Stir in chicken, arugula and tomatoes.

- Top with pine nuts. Serve at room temperature or refrigerate until cold, about 2 hours.

Edamame & Chicken Greek Salad

Ingredients

- 1 8-ounce boneless skinless chicken breast, trimmed
- ¼ cup red-wine vinegar
- 3 tablespoons extra-virgin olive oil
- ¼ teaspoon salt
- ¼ teaspoon ground pepper
- 8 ounces frozen shelled edamame (about 1 1/2 cups), thawed
- 8 cups chopped romaine (about 2 romaine hearts)
- 1 cup halved cherry or grape tomatoes
- ½ European cucumber, sliced
- ½ cup crumbled feta cheese
- ¼ cup slivered fresh basil
- ¼ cup sliced Kalamata olives
- ¼ cup slivered red onion

Directions

- Place chicken in a medium saucepan and add water to cover by 2 inches. Bring to a boil. Reduce heat to a simmer and cook until an instant-read thermometer inserted into the chicken registers 165 degrees F, 12 to 15 minutes. Transfer the chicken to a clean cutting board and let cool for 5 minutes; shred or chop into bite-size pieces.
- Meanwhile, whisk vinegar, oil, salt and pepper in a large bowl. Add edamame,

romaine, tomatoes, cucumber, feta, basil, olives, onion and the chicken; toss to coat.

Tomato, Cucumber & White-Bean Salad with Basil Vinaigrette

Ingredients

- ½ cup packed fresh basil leaves
- ¼ cup extra-virgin olive oil
- 3 tablespoons red-wine vinegar
- 1 tablespoon finely chopped shallot
- 2 teaspoons Dijon mustard
- 1 teaspoon honey
- ¼ teaspoon salt
- ¼ teaspoon ground pepper
- 10 cups mixed salad greens
- 1 (15 ounce) can low-sodium cannellini beans, rinsed
- 1 cup halved cherry or grape tomatoes
- ½ cucumber, halved lengthwise and sliced (1 cup)

Directions

Step 1

Place basil, oil, vinegar, shallot, mustard, honey, salt and pepper in a mini food processor. Process until mostly smooth. Transfer to a large bowl. Add greens, beans, tomatoes and cucumber. Toss to coat.

Couscous & Chickpea Salad

Ingredients

- 1 cup finely chopped kale
- ¾ cup cooked whole-wheat couscous
- ⅔ cup rinsed canned chickpeas
- 4 tablespoons Basil Vinaigrette

Directions

- Combine kale, couscous, chickpeas and dressing in a medium bowl. Serve immediately or refrigerate in a sealable container for up to 4 days.

Meal-Prep Roasted Vegetable Bowls with Pesto

Ingredients

- 3 tablespoons extra-virgin olive oil, divided
- ½ teaspoon garlic powder
- ¼ teaspoon salt
- ¼ teaspoon ground pepper
- 4 cups broccoli florets
- 2 medium red bell peppers, quartered
- 1 cup sliced red onion
- 3 cups cooked brown rice
- 1 (15 ounce) can chickpeas, rinsed
- 4 tablespoons prepared pesto

Directions

- Preheat oven to 450 degrees F.
- Whisk 2 tablespoons oil, garlic powder, salt and pepper together in a large bowl. Add broccoli, peppers and onion; toss to coat. Transfer to a large rimmed baking sheet and roast, stirring once, until the vegetables are tender, about 20 minutes. Chop the peppers when cool enough to handle.
- Stir the remaining 1 tablespoon oil into rice. Place about 3/4 cup of the rice in each of four 2-cup microwave-safe,

lidded containers. Divide chickpeas and the roasted vegetables among the bowls. Top each with 1 tablespoon pesto.

- To reheat: Microwave each container on High until heated through, 1 to 2 minutes.

Beet & Shrimp Winter Salad

Ingredients

- Salad
- 2 cups lightly packed arugula
- 1 cup lightly packed watercress
- 1 cup cooked beet wedges
- ½ cup zucchini ribbons (see Tip)
- ½ cup thinly sliced fennel
- ½ cup cooked barley
- 4 ounces cooked, peeled shrimp (see Tip), tails left on if desired
- Fennel fronds for garnish
- Vinaigrette
- 2 tablespoons extra-virgin olive oil
- 1 tablespoon red- or white-wine vinegar
- ½ teaspoon Dijon mustard
- ½ teaspoon minced shallot
- ¼ teaspoon ground pepper
- ⅛ teaspoon salt

Directions

- Arrange arugula, watercress, beets, zucchini, fennel, barley and shrimp on a large dinner plate.
- Whisk oil, vinegar, mustard, shallot, pepper and salt in a small bowl, then drizzle over the salad. Garnish with fennel fronds, if desired.

Creamy Pesto Chicken Salad with Greens

Ingredients

- 1 pound boneless, skinless chicken breast, trimmed
- ¼ cup pesto
- ¼ cup low-fat mayonnaise
- 3 tablespoons finely chopped red onion
- 2 tablespoons extra-virgin olive oil
- 2 tablespoons red-wine vinegar
- ¼ teaspoon salt
- ¼ teaspoon ground pepper
- 1 5-ounce package mixed salad greens (about 8 cups)
- 1 pint grape or cherry tomatoes, halved

Directions

- Place chicken in a medium saucepan and add water to cover by 1 inch. Bring to a boil. Cover, reduce heat to low and simmer gently until no longer pink in the middle, 10 to 15 minutes. Transfer to a clean cutting board; shred into bite-size pieces when cool enough to handle.
- Combine pesto, mayonnaise and onion in a medium bowl. Add the chicken and toss to coat. Whisk oil, vinegar, salt and pepper in a large bowl. Add greens and tomatoes and toss to coat. Divide the green salad among 4 plates and top with the chicken salad.

Tabbouleh, Hummus & Pita Plate

Ingredients

- 2 cups tabbouleh
- 1 cup beet hummus
- 1 cup sugar snap peas, stem ends snapped off
- 4 radishes
- 1 cup mixed olives
- 1 cup raspberries
- 1 cup blackberries
- 4 (4 inch) whole-wheat pita breads
- ⅔ cup unsalted dry-roasted pistachios
- 4 vegan cookies

Directions

- Divide items equally among 4 plates.

Mediterranean Edamame Toss

Ingredients

- ½ cup uncooked quinoa, rinsed and drained
- 1 cup water
- 1 cup ready-to-eat fresh or frozen, thawed shelled sweet soybeans (edamame)
- 2 medium tomatoes, seeded and chopped
- 1 cup fresh arugula or spinach leaves
- ½ cup chopped red onion
- 2 tablespoons olive oil
- 1 teaspoon finely shredded lemon peel
- 2 tablespoons lemon juice
- ¼ cup crumbled reduced-fat feta cheese
- 2 tablespoons snipped fresh basil
- ¼ teaspoon salt
- ¼ teaspoon freshly ground black pepper

Directions

- In a medium saucepan, combine quinoa and water. Bring to boiling; reduce heat. Cover and simmer about 15 minutes or until quinoa is tender and liquid is absorbed, adding edamame the last 4 minutes of cooking.
- In a large bowl, combine quinoa mixture, tomato, arugula, and onion.
- In a small bowl, whisk together olive oil, lemon peel, and lemon juice. Stir in half of the cheese, the basil, salt, and pepper. Add mixture to quinoa mixture, tossing to coat. Sprinkle with remaining half of the cheese. Serve at room temperature.

Fig & Goat Cheese Salad

Ingredients

- 2 cups mixed salad greens
- 4 dried figs, stemmed and sliced
- 1 ounce fresh goat cheese, crumbled
- 1 ½ tablespoons slivered almonds, preferably toasted
- 2 teaspoons extra-virgin olive oil
- 2 teaspoons balsamic vinegar
- ½ teaspoon honey
- Pinch of salt
- Freshly ground pepper to taste

Directions

- Combine greens, figs, goat cheese and almonds in a medium bowl. Stir together oil, vinegar, honey, salt and pepper.
- Just before serving, drizzle the dressing over the salad and toss.

White Bean & Veggie Salad

Ingredients

- 2 cups mixed salad greens
- ¾ cup veggies of your choice, such as chopped cucumbers and cherry tomatoes
- ⅓ cup canned white beans, rinsed and drained
- ½ avocado, diced
- 1 tablespoon red-wine vinegar
- 2 teaspoons extra-virgin olive oil
- ¼ teaspoon kosher salt
- Freshly ground pepper to taste

Directions

- Combine greens, veggies, beans and avocado in a medium bowl. Drizzle with vinegar and oil and season with salt and pepper. Toss to combine and transfer to a large plate.

Greek-Style Chicken Salad

Ingredients

- 2 cups Shredded Chicken Master Recipe
- ½ cup bottled reduced-calorie Greek vinaigrette salad dressing, divided
- 1 teaspoon finely shredded lemon zest
- ½ teaspoon dried oregano, crushed
- 6 cups torn romaine lettuce
- 1 ½ cups chopped cucumber (1 medium)
- 1 cup grape tomatoes, halved
- ¾ cup chopped yellow sweet pepper (1 medium)
- ½ cup thinly sliced red onion, rings separated
- ½ cup crumbled reduced-fat feta cheese (2 ounces)
- ¼ cup pitted Kalamata olives, halved
- 4 Lemon wedges for garnish

Directions

- In a medium bowl, combine chicken, 1/4 cup vinaigrette, lemon zest and oregano; set aside.
- Meanwhile, in a large salad bowl, toss lettuce with the remaining 1/4 cup vinaigrette. Spoon 1 1/2 cups lettuce into each of four shallow bowls. Top each with about 1/3 cup cucumber, 1/4 cup tomatoes, 3 tablespoons sweet pepper, and 2 tablespoons onion. Add chicken mixture to the center of each. Sprinkle with 2 tablespoons feta and 1 tablespoon olives. If desired, serve with lemon wedges.

Quinoa Chickpea Salad with Roasted Red Pepper Hummus Dressing

Ingredients

- 2 tablespoons hummus, original or roasted red pepper flavor
- 1 tablespoon lemon juice
- 1 tablespoon chopped roasted red pepper
- 2 cups mixed salad greens
- ½ cup cooked quinoa
- ½ cup chickpeas, rinsed
- 1 tablespoon unsalted sunflower seeds
- 1 tablespoon chopped fresh parsley

- Pinch of salt
- Pinch of ground pepper

Directions

- Stir hummus, lemon juice and red peppers in a small dish. Thin with water to desired consistency for dressing.
- Arrange greens, quinoa and chickpeas in a large bowl. Top with sunflower seeds, parsley, salt and pepper. Serve with the dressing.

Meal-Prep Falafel Bowls with Tahini Sauce

Ingredients

- 1 (8 ounce) package frozen prepared falafel
- ⅔ cup water
- ½ cup whole-wheat couscous
- 1 (16 ounce) bag steam-in-bag fresh green beans
- 1/2 cup Tahini Sauce (see associated recipe)
- ¼ cup pitted Kalamata olives
- ¼ cup crumbled feta cheese

Directions

- Prepare falafel according to package directions; set aside to cool.
- Bring water to a boil in a small saucepan. Stir in couscous, cover and remove from heat. Allow to stand until the liquid is absorbed, about 5 minutes. Fluff with a fork; set aside.
- Prepare green beans according to package directions.
- Prepare Tahini Sauce. Divide among 4 small condiment containers with lids and refrigerate.
- Divide the green beans among 4 single-serving containers with lids. Top each with 1/2 cup couscous, one-fourth of the falafel and 1 tablespoon each olives and feta. Seal and refrigerate for up to 4 days.
- To serve, reheat in the microwave until heated through, about 2 minutes. Dress with tahini sauce just before eating.

Shrimp, Avocado & Feta Wrap

Ingredients

- 3 ounces chopped cooked shrimp
- ¼ cup diced avocado
- ¼ cup diced tomato
- 1 scallion, sliced
- 2 tablespoons crumbled feta cheese
- 1 tablespoon lime juice
- 1 whole-wheat tortilla

Directions

- Combine shrimp, avocado, tomato, scallion, feta and lime juice in a small bowl. Serve in tortilla.

Mediterranean Veggie Wrap with Cilantro Hummus

Ingredients

Cilantro Hummus

- 1 clove garlic, peeled
- 1 (15 ounce) can no-salt-added garbanzo beans (chickpeas)

- 3 tablespoons lemon juice
- 2 tablespoons olive oil
- 1 tablespoon tahini (sesame seed paste)
- ¼ teaspoon salt
- ¼ teaspoon white pepper
- ¼ cup fresh cilantro leaves

Mediterranean Wraps

- 4 cups mixed baby greens
- ½ large cucumber, halved lengthwise and sliced (1 cup)
- 1 cup chopped tomato
- ½ cup thinly sliced red onion
- ¼ cup crumbled reduced-fat feta cheese
- 2 tablespoons bottled sliced mild banana peppers
- 1 tablespoon balsamic vinegar
- 1 tablespoon olive oil
- 1 clove garlic, minced
- ¼ teaspoon black pepper
- 4 (8 inch) light tomato-flavored oval multi-grain wraps

Directions

- To prepare Cilantro Hummus: With the motor running, drop 1 clove peeled garlic through the feed tube of a food processor fitted with a steel blade attachment; process until finely minced. Scrape down the sides of the bowl. Rinse and drain one 15-ounce can no-salt-added garbanzo beans (chickpeas). Add garbanzo beans, 3 tablespoons lemon juice, 2 tablespoons olive oil, 1 tablespoon tahini (sesame seed paste), 1/4 teaspoon salt and 1/4 teaspoon white pepper. Process until completely smooth,

stopping to scrape down the sides as necessary. Add 1/4 cup fresh cilantro leaves. Pulse several times or until cilantro is evenly distributed and chopped. Chill until ready to use (see Tip).

- To prepare Mediterranean Wraps: In a large bowl combine greens, cucumber, tomato, red onion, feta cheese and banana peppers. In a small bowl whisk together vinegar, olive oil, garlic and black pepper. Pour dressing mixture over greens mixture. Toss to combine.

- Spread each wrap with about 2 1/2 tablespoons hummus. Top with dressed greens mixture. Roll up. Serve immediately.

Vegan Bistro Lunch Box

Ingredients

- ¼ cup hummus
- ½ whole-wheat pita bread, cut into 4 wedges
- 2 tablespoons mixed olives
- 1 Persian cucumber or 1/2 English cucumber, cut into spears
- ¼ large red bell pepper, sliced
- ¼ teaspoon chopped fresh dill

Directions

- Arrange hummus, pita, olives, cucumber and bell peppers in a 4-cup divided sealable container. (If desired, the hummus and olives can be kept separate by placing them in silicone baking cups before arranging.) Sprinkle cucumber with dill. Keep refrigerated until ready to use.

Mediterranean Chicken Salad

Ingredients

- ⅓ cup lemon juice
- 2 tablespoons snipped fresh mint
- 2 tablespoons snipped fresh basil
- 2 tablespoons olive oil
- 1 tablespoon honey
- ¼ teaspoon ground black pepper
- 5 cups shredded romaine lettuce
- 2 cups cut-up cooked chicken breast
- 2 plum tomatoes, cut into wedges
- 1 (15 ounce) can garbanzo beans (chickpeas), rinsed and drained
- 2 tablespoons pitted Kalamata olives, quartered (Optional)
- 2 tablespoons crumbled reduced-fat feta cheese
- 6 Whole kalamata olives for garnish (Optional)

Directions

- In a screw-top jar, combine lemon juice, mint, basil, olive oil, honey, and black pepper to make dressing. Cover and shake well.
- Place lettuce on a large platter. Top with chicken, tomatoes, garbanzo beans, the quartered olives (if using), and feta cheese. Drizzle with dressing. If desired, garnish individual servings with whole olives.

Edamame Hummus Wrap

Ingredients

- 12 ounces frozen shelled edamame (about 2 1/4 cups), thawed
- 4 tablespoons lemon juice, divided
- 3 tablespoons extra-virgin olive oil, divided
- 2 tablespoons tahini
- 1 large clove garlic, chopped
- ½ teaspoon ground cumin
- ¾ teaspoon ground pepper, divided
- ½ teaspoon salt
- 2 cups very thinly sliced green cabbage
- ½ cup sliced orange bell pepper
- 1 scallion, thinly sliced
- ¼ cup chopped fresh parsley
- 4 8- to 9-inch spinach or whole-wheat tortillas

Directions

- Combine edamame, 3 tablespoons lemon juice, 2 tablespoons oil, tahini, garlic, cumin, 1/2 teaspoon pepper and salt in a food processor. Pulse until fairly smooth.
- Whisk the remaining 1 tablespoon each lemon juice and oil with the remaining 1/4 teaspoon pepper in a medium bowl. Add cabbage, bell pepper, scallion and parsley; toss to coat. Spread about 1/2 cup of the edamame hummus across the lower third of each tortilla and top with about 1/2 cup of the cabbage mixture. Roll closed. Cut in half to serve, if desired.

Tomato Salad with Grilled Halloumi and Herbs

INGREDIENTS

- 1 pound tomatoes, sliced into rounds
- ½ lemon
- Flaky salt and freshly ground pepper
- Extra-virgin olive oil
- ½ pound halloumi cheese, sliced into 4 slabs
- 5 basil leaves, torn
- 2 tablespoons finely chopped flat-leaf parsley

DIRECTIONS

- Preheat a grill or grill pan over medium-high heat.
- Arrange the tomatoes on a serving platter or four plates. Lightly squeeze the lemon over them and season with flaky salt and pepper.
- Brush the grill grates with oil, then add the halloumi and cook, turning once, until marks appear and the cheese is warmed throughout, about 1 minute per side. Place on top of the tomatoes. Drizzle the salad with olive oil and sprinkle with the basil and parsley. Serve immediately.

Harissa Chickpea Stew with Eggplant and Millet

INGREDIENTS

- 1 cup millet
- 2 tablespoons harissa paste
- 1 bunch cilantro, for garnish
- Kosher salt
- 2 tablespoons ghee (or another neutral high-heat oil), divided
- 1 large Japanese eggplant
- Freshly ground black pepper
- 1 onion, diced
- 3 garlic cloves, minced
- One fourteen-ounce can pureed tomatoes

DIRECTIONS

- Fill a medium saucepan with 2 cups water and add the millet and a pinch of salt. Bring to a boil, cover, reduce to a simmer and cook for 25 minutes. Once the millet is done cooking, remove the lid, fluff with a fork and allow to cool.
- Meanwhile, heat 1 tablespoon of ghee or oil in a deep skillet over medium heat. Add the eggplant, season with salt and pepper, and cook until tender and golden brown, adding more ghee as necessary to prevent the eggplant from sticking to the skillet, about 10 minutes. Transfer the eggplant to a bowl and set it aside.
- Add the remaining 1 tablespoon of ghee or oil to the same skillet, add the onion and cook until soft and golden brown, 8 to 10 minutes.
- Add the garlic and cook for 2 more minutes. Season with salt and pepper, and then add the tomatoes, chickpeas and harissa. Return the eggplant to the skillet and reduce the heat to low; allow to simmer for 10 to 15 minutes.

- Divide the millet between two bowls and top with the stew. Garnish with a few leaves of cilantro and serve warm.

Grilled Lemon-Herb Chicken and Avocado Salad

- 1½ pounds boneless, skinless chicken breasts
- 3 tablespoons extra-virgin olive oil
- Zest and juice of 2 lemons
- 1 tablespoon chopped fresh oregano
- 1 tablespoon chopped fresh dill
- 3 tablespoons chopped fresh parsley
- Kosher salt and freshly ground black pepper

SALAD

- 1 cup barley
- 2½ cups chicken broth
- Zest and juice of 1 lemon
- 1 tablespoon whole-grain mustard
- 1 teaspoon dried oregano
- ⅓ cup extra-virgin olive oil
- Kosher salt and freshly ground black pepper
- 2 heads red-leaf lettuce, chopped
- 1 red onion, halved and thinly sliced
- 1 pint cherry tomatoes, sliced
- 2 avocados, sliced

Directions

- **MAKE THE LEMON-HERB CHICKEN:** Place the chicken in a large resealable plastic bag. In a medium bowl, whisk together the olive oil, lemon zest, lemon juice, oregano, dill and parsley. Pour the marinade into the bag, seal it and refrigerate for 30 minutes.
- **MAKE THE SALAD:** Meanwhile, in a medium saucepan, bring the barley and chicken broth to a simmer over medium heat. When it comes to a simmer, cover the pot and cook until the barley is tender, 35 to 45 minutes. Drain and reserve.
- In a medium bowl, whisk together the lemon zest, lemon juice, mustard and oregano. Gradually stream in the olive oil and whisk well to combine. Season with salt and pepper.
- Prepare your grill for high heat. Remove the chicken from the marinade and season with salt and pepper.
- Grill the chicken until well charred on both sides and fully cooked through, flipping as needed, 10 to 12 minutes. Remove the chicken from the grill and reserve.
- In a large bowl, toss together the lettuce, onion and tomatoes. Add the dressing and toss well to coat.
- Slice the chicken and serve on top of the salad alongside the avocado.

5-Minute Heirloom Tomato and Cucumber Toast

- 1 small heirloom tomato, diced
- 1 Persian cucumber, diced
- 1 teaspoon extra-virgin olive oil
- Pinch of dried oregano

- Kosher salt and freshly ground black pepper
- 2 teaspoons low-fat whipped cream cheese
- 2 pieces Trader Joe's Whole Grain Crispbread
- 1 teaspoon balsamic glaze

Directions

- In a medium bowl, combine the tomato, cucumber, olive oil and oregano; season with salt and pepper.
- Smear the cream cheese on the bread and top with the tomato-cucumber mixture and the balsamic glaze.

Greek Chicken and Rice Skillet

- 6 chicken thighs
- Kosher salt and freshly ground black pepper
- 1 teaspoon dried oregano
- 1 teaspoon garlic powder
- 3 lemons
- 2 tablespoons extra-virgin olive oil
- ½ red onion, minced
- 2 garlic cloves, minced
- 1 cup long-grain rice
- 2½ cups chicken broth
- 1 tablespoon chopped fresh oregano, plus more for garnishing
- 1 cup green olives
- ½ cup crumbled feta cheese
- ⅓ cup fresh chopped fresh parsley

Directions

- Preheat the oven to 375°F. Season the chicken thighs with salt and pepper. In a small bowl, stir together the dried oregano, garlic powder and the zest of 1 lemon. Rub the mixture evenly over the chicken.
- Heat the olive oil in a large oven-safe skillet over medium heat. Add the chicken, skin side down, and sear until the chicken is well browned, 7 to 9 minutes. Remove to a plate and reserve.
- Add the onion and garlic to the skillet and sauté until translucent, about 5 minutes. Stir in the rice and sauté for 1 minute; season with salt.
- Add the chicken broth and bring the mixture to a simmer. Stir in the fresh oregano and the juice of the zested lemon. Slice the remaining 2 lemons and set aside.
- Nestle the chicken, skin side up, into the rice mixture. Transfer the skillet to the oven and cook until the rice has absorbed all of the liquid and the chicken is fully cooked, 20 to 25 minutes.
- Turn on the broiler and arrange the lemon slices over the chicken. Broil the skillet until the lemons are lightly charred and the chicken skin is very crisp, about 3 minutes.
- Add the olives and feta to the skillet, garnish with fresh parsley and serve immediately.

Mini Chicken Shawarma

CHICKEN

- 1 pound chicken tenders
- ¼ cup extra-virgin olive oil
- Zest and juice of 1 lemon
- 2 teaspoons garlic powder
- 1 teaspoon ground cumin
- ¾ teaspoon ground coriander
- ½ teaspoon smoked paprika
- 1 teaspoon freshly ground black pepper

SAUCE

- 1¼ cups Greek yogurt
- 1 tablespoon lemon juice
- 1 garlic clove, grated
- ¼ cup chopped fresh parsley
- 2 tablespoons chopped fresh dill
- Kosher salt and freshly ground black pepper
- ½ red onion, thinly sliced
- 4 leaves romaine lettuce, shredded
- ½ English cucumber, thinly sliced
- 2 tomatoes, chopped
- 16 mini pita breads

Directions

- **MAKE THE CHICKEN:** Place the chicken in a large resealable plastic bag. In a small bowl, whisk together the olive oil, lemon zest, lemon juice, garlic powder, cumin, coriander, paprika and pepper to combine. Pour the marinade into the bag, seal and toss the chicken well to coat. Let the chicken marinate for 30 minutes to 1 hour.
- **MAKE THE SAUCE:** While the chicken marinates, stir together the Greek yogurt, lemon juice and garlic in a medium bowl.

Stir in the parsley and dill; season with salt and pepper. Cover and refrigerate.

- Heat a large skillet over medium heat. Remove the chicken from the marinade, letting the excess drip off, and cook until it's well browned on both sides and fully cooked, about 4 minutes per side. Chop it into bite-size strips.
- To assemble, divide the chicken, onion, lettuce, cucumber and tomato

Mediterranean feta salad with pomegranate dressing

Ingredients

- 2 red peppers
- 3medium aubergines , cut into chunks, or 15 small, halved
- 6 tbsp extra-virgin olive oil
- tsp cinnamon
- 200g green bean , blanched (use frozen if you can)
- 1 small red onion , sliced into half moons
- 200g feta cheese , drained and crumbled
- seeds 1 pomegranate
- handful parsley , roughly chopped
- For the dressing
- 1 small garlic clove , crushed
- 1 tbsp lemon juice
- 2 tbsp pomegranate molasses
- 5 tbsp extra-virgin olive oil

Method

- Heat oven to 200C/fan 180C/gas 6. Heat the grill to its highest setting. Cut the peppers into quarters, then place them, skin-side up, on a baking sheet. Grill until blackened. Place in a plastic bag, seal, then leave for 5 mins. When cool enough to handle, scrape skins off, discard, then set the peppers aside.

- Place the aubergines on a baking tray, drizzle with olive oil and cinnamon, then season with salt and pepper. Roast until golden and softened – about 25 mins.
- Meanwhile, combine all the dressing ingredients and mix well. To serve, place the aubergines, green beans, onion and peppers on a large serving plate. Scatter with the feta and pomegranate seeds. Pour the dressing over, then finish with the parsley.

Mediterranean scones

Ingredients

- 350g self-raising flour
- 1 tbsp baking powder
- ¼ tsp salt
- 50g butter , cut in pieces
- 1 tbsp olive oil
- 8 halves Italian sundried tomatoes , coarsely chopped
- 100g feta cheese , cubed
- 10 black olives , pitted and halved
- 300ml full fat milk
- 1 egg , beaten, to glaze

Method

- Heat the oven to 220C/fan 200C/gas 7. Butter a large baking sheet. In a large bowl, mix together the flour, baking powder and salt. Rub in the butter with the oil, until the mixture resembles fine crumbs, then add the tomatoes, cheese and olives. Make a well in the centre, pour in the milk and mix with a knife, using a cutting movement, until it becomes a soft 'stickyish' dough. (Use all the milk – it helps give a light texture.) Don't overhandle the dough.
- Flour your hands and the work surface well, and shape the dough into a round, about 3-4cm thick. Cut into eight wedges and place them well apart on the baking sheet. Brush with beaten egg and bake for 15-20 mins until risen, golden and springy to the touch. Transfer to a wire rack and cover with a clean tea towel to keep them soft. These are best served warm and buttered. Will keep for 2-3 days in an airtight container.

Spiced baked figs with ginger mascarpone

Ingredients

- 8 figs , halved
- 2 tbsp butter
- 2 tbsp clear honey
- 2 tbsp brown sugar
- 2 tsp ground cinnamon
- 2 tbsp orange juice
- 2 star anise
- shortbread fingers, to serve
- For the ginger mascarpone
- 1 ball stem ginger , very finely chopped
- 1 tbsp ginger syrup from the jar
- ½ a 250g tub mascarpone

Method

- Heat oven to 200C/180C fan/gas 6. Lay the figs in an ovenproof roasting dish, dot over the butter and drizzle with honey. Sprinkle over the sugar and cinnamon, then pour over the orange juice and mix lightly. Nestle the star anise amongst the figs and roast for 15-20 minutes.
- When ready to serve, mix the ginger and syrup through the mascarpone. Place 4 fig halves, drizzled with syrup, on a plate with a dollop of mascarpone and some shortbread fingers.

Crispy squid with caponata

Ingredients

- 800g cleaned squid tubes (about 3 large tubes)
- 150g plain flour
- 1 tbsp cayenne pepper or chilli powder
- sunflower oil , for frying
- For the caponata
- 1 large aubergine
- 4 tbsp extra-virgin olive oil
- 1 onion , chopped
- 3 celery sticks, sliced
- 250g cherry tomatoes
- 3 garlic cloves , crushed
- 1 tsp caster sugar
- 1 tbsp balsamic vinegar
- 150g green olive , stoned
- 30g caper , rinsed if salted
- handful basil leaves, shredded

Method

- To prepare the squid, lay the squid flat on a board. Insert a long, thin knife in the opening and neatly cut it along one side. Open it out to a flat sheet and scrape away any leftover membrane. Use the tip of the knife to lightly score the flesh in a diamond pattern, taking care not to cut through the squid completely. Cut the scored squid into large triangles ready to be floured and fried.
- For the caponata, the aubergine needs to be cut into uniform dice: slice it lengthways about 1cm thick, cut long strips the same size, then chop them into squares.
- Heat half the oil in a large sauté pan. Fry the onions for 3-4 mins until starting to soften, add the aubergine, then continue to cook for 8-10 mins until brown and soft. Tip into a colander over a bowl.
- Tip any oil from the bowl back into the pan and top it up with a splash of fresh oil. Fry the celery, tomatoes and the crushed garlic together. Sprinkle the sugar over, splash in the vinegar, then cook for 3-4 mins until the tomatoes start to release their juice.
- Tip the aubergine and onion back in with the celery. Scatter in the olives, capers and basil, then give everything a good stir. Cook for 5 mins until simmering, then season to taste. Turn off the heat, drizzle in the rest of the oil, then set aside.
- Just before cooking, tip the squid into a large bowl. Sift the flour and cayenne pepper together over the squid, then toss well and season with salt. Tip the squid

back into the sieve and shake off all the excess flour.

- Pour enough sunflower oil into a large frying pan so it's about 1cm deep. Heat the oil until it sizzles when sprinkled with a little flour. In batches, fry the squid for 2-3 mins on each side until golden and crisp. When cooked, use tongs to lift the squid onto a plate lined with kitchen paper. You are now ready to serve.

- Spoon the caponata inside a 10cm wide metal ring (or simply make a neat pile) in the middle of a medium dinner plate. Use the back of the spoon to press down lightly on the caponata and level the top of the pile. Carefully lift the ring away, keeping the tower of caponata circular. Lean five or six pieces of squid around the caponata like petals on a flower, then serve immediately.

Watermelon & feta salad with crispbread

Ingredients

- ½ a watermelon (about 1.5kg), peeled, deseeded and cut into chunks
- 200g block feta cheese , cubed
- large handful black olives
- handful flat-leaf parsley and mint leaves, roughly chopped
- 1 red onion , finely sliced into rings
- olive oil and balsamic vinegar, to serve

For the crispbread

- ½ a 500g pack white bread mix

- 1 tbsp olive oil , plus a little extra for drizzling
- plain flour , for dusting
- 1 egg white , beaten
- a mix of sesame seeds , poppy seeds and fennel seeds, for scattering

Method

- Make up the bread according to pack instructions with 1 tbsp olive oil. Leave to rise in a warm place for about 1 hr until doubled in size. Heat oven to 220C/200C fan/gas 7. Knock the bread back and divide into 6 pieces. On a floured surface, roll the breads out as thinly as possible, then transfer to baking trays. Brush with the egg white and scatter with the mixed seeds. Bake for about 15 mins until crisp and brown; if they puff up, even better. You may need to do this in batches. The breads can be made the previous day and kept in an airtight container.

- In a large serving bowl, lightly toss the melon with the feta and olives. Scatter over the herbs and onion rings, then serve with the olive oil and balsamic for drizzling over. Serve the pile of crispbreads on the side for breaking up and using to scoop the salad.

Aïoli

Ingredients

- small pinch saffron strands
- 3 garlic cloves , crushed
- 2 egg yolks

- 1 tbsp Dijon mustard
- 300ml olive oil

Method

- In a small bowl pour 1 tbsp of boiling water over the saffron and set aside.
- Put the garlic, egg yolks and mustard into a food processor or blender.
- Blitz into a paste and very slowly dribble in the olive oil to make a thick mayonnaise-style sauce.
- When everything's come together add the saffron, saffron water and lemon juice, then season to taste. The aïoli will keep covered in the fridge for up to 2 days.

Crunchy baked mussels

Ingredients

- 1kg mussel in their shells
- 50g toasted breadcrumb
- zest 1 lemon
- 100g garlic and parsley butter

Method

- Scrub the mussels and pull off any beards. Rinse in several changes of cold water, then discard any that are open and do not close when tapped against the side of the sink.
- Drain the mussels and put in a large pan with a splash of water. Bring to the boil, then cover the pan, shaking occasionally, until the mussels are open – this will take 2-3 mins. Drain well, then discard any that remain closed. Heat grill to high.

- Mix the crumbs and zest. Remove one side of each shell, then spread a little butter onto each mussel. Set on a baking tray and sprinkle with crumbs. Grill for 3-4 mins until crunchy.

Easy stuffed peppers

Ingredients

- 4 red peppers
- 2 x pouches cooked tomato rice (we used Tilda Rizazz Mediterranean Tomato)
- 2 tbsp pesto
- handful pitted black olives, chopped
- 200g goat's cheese, sliced

Method

- Use a small knife to cut the top out of 4 red peppers, then scoop out the seeds. Sit the peppers on a plate, cut-side up, and cook in the microwave on High for 5-6 mins until they have wilted and softened.
- While the peppers are cooking, mix two 250g pouches cooked tomato rice together with 2 tbsp pesto and a handful of chopped pitted black olives and 140g of the sliced goat's cheese.
- Scoop the rice, pesto, olives and goat's cheese mix into the peppers, top with the remaining 60g sliced goat's cheese and continue to cook for 8-10 mins.

Mediterranean slices

Ingredients

- 375g pack ready-rolled puff pastry

- 4 tbsp green pesto
- 140g frozen sliced roasted peppers
- 140g frozen artichokes (about 3 wedges per serving)
- 125g ball mozzarella , or 85g cheddar, grated

Method

- Heat oven to 200C/fan 180C/gas 6. Unroll the pastry and cut into 4 rectangles. Take a sharp knife and score a 1cm edge inside each rectangle, taking care that you don't cut all the way through the pastry. Place on a baking sheet.
- Spread 1 tbsp pesto onto each slice, staying inside the border, then pile up the peppers and artichokes. Cook in the oven for 15 mins until the pastry is starting to brown.
- Tear the mozzarella ball into small pieces, then scatter it (or use cheddar, if you prefer) over the veg. Return to the oven for 5-7 mins until the pastry is crisp and the cheese has melted. Serve with a green salad.

Mediterranean chicken tray bake

Ingredients

- 2 red peppers , deseeded and cut into chunks
- 1 red onion , cut into wedges
- 2 tsp olive oil
- 4 skin-on chicken breasts

- ½ x 150g pack full-fat garlic & herb soft cheese
- 200g pack cherry tomatoes
- handful black olives

Method

- Heat oven to 200C/180C fan/gas 6. Mix the peppers and onion on a big baking tray with half the oil. Transfer to the oven and cook on the top shelf for 10 mins.
- Meanwhile, carefully make a pocket between the skin and the flesh of each chicken breast, but don't pull off the skin completely. Push equal amounts of cheese under the skin, smooth the skin back down, brush it with the rest of the oil, season, then add to the tray along with the tomatoes and olives. Return to the oven and cook for 25-30 mins more until the chicken is golden and cooked. Serve with baked potatoes, if you like.

Mussels with tomatoes & chilli

Ingredients

- 2 ripe tomatoes
- 2 tbsp olive oil
- 1 garlic clove , finely chopped
- 1 shallot , finely chopped
- 1 red or green chilli , deseeded and finely chopped
- small glass dry white wine
- 1 tsp tomato paste
- pinch of sugar
- 1kg cleaned mussels
- good handful basil leaves

Method

- Put the tomatoes in a heatproof bowl. Cover with boiling water, leave for 3 mins, then drain and peel. Quarter the tomatoes and scoop out and discard the seeds using a teaspoon. Roughly chop the tomato flesh.
- Heat the oil in a large pan with a tight-fitting lid. Add the garlic, shallot and chilli, then gently fry for 2-3 mins until softened. Pour in the wine and add the tomatoes, paste, sugar and seasoning (mussels are naturally salty so take care with the salt). Stir well and simmer for 2 mins.
- Tip in the mussels and give them a stir. Cover tightly and steam for 3-4 mins, shaking the pan halfway through, until the shells have opened.
- Discard any shells that remain shut, then divide the mussels between two bowls and add the basil leaves. Provide a large bowl for the empty shells.

Mediterranean chicken with roasted vegetables

Ingredients

- 250g baby new potatoes, thinly sliced
- 1 large courgette, diagonally sliced
- 1 red onion, cut into wedges
- 1 yellow pepper, seeded and cut into chunks
- 6 firm plum tomatoes, halved
- 12 black olives, pitted
- 2 skinless boneless chicken breast fillets, about 150g/5oz each
- 3 tbsp olive oil
- 1 rounded tbsp green pesto

Method

- Preheat the oven to 200C/ Gas 6/fan oven 180C. Spread the potatoes, courgette, onion, pepper and tomatoes in a shallow roasting tin and scatter over the olives. Season with salt and coarsely ground black pepper.
- Slash the flesh of each chicken breast 3-4 times using a sharp knife, then lay the chicken on top of the vegetables.
- Mix the olive oil and pesto together until well blended and spoon evenly over the chicken. Cover the tin with foil and cook for 30 minutes.
- Remove the foil from the tin. Return to the oven and cook for a further 10 minutes until the vegetables are juicy and look tempting to eat and the chicken is cooked through (the juices should run clear when pierced with a skewer).

Roasted peppers with tomatoes & anchovies

Ingredients

- 4 red peppers , halved and deseeded
- 50g can anchovy in oil, drained
- 8 smallish tomatoes , halved
- 2 garlic cloves , thinly sliced
- 2 rosemary sprigs
- 2 tbsp olive oil

Method

- Heat oven to 160C/140C fan/gas 3. Put the peppers into a large baking dish, toss with a little of the oil from the anchovy can, then turn cut-side up. Roast for 40 mins, until soft but not collapsed.

- Slice 8 of the anchovies along their length. Put 2 halves of tomato, several garlic slices, a few little rosemary sprigs and two pieces of anchovy into the hollow of each pepper. Drizzle over the olive oil, then roast again for 30 mins until the tomatoes are soft and the peppers are filled with pools of tasty juice. Leave to cool and serve warm or at room temperature.

MEDITERRANEAN LUNCH RECIPE

Mediterranean Stuffed Chicken Breasts

Ingredients

- ½ cup crumbled feta cheese
- ½ cup chopped roasted red bell peppers
- ½ cup chopped fresh spinach
- ¼ cup Kalamata olives, pitted and quartered
- 1 tablespoon chopped fresh basil
- 1 tablespoon chopped fresh flat-leaf parsley
- 2 cloves garlic, minced
- 4 (8 ounce) boneless, skinless chicken breasts
- ¼ teaspoon salt
- ½ teaspoon ground pepper

- 1 tablespoon extra-virgin olive oil
- 1 tablespoon lemon juice

Directions

- Preheat oven to 400 degrees F. Combine feta, roasted red peppers, spinach, olives, basil, parsley and garlic in a medium bowl.

- Using a small knife, cut a horizontal slit through the thickest portion of each chicken breast to form a pocket. Stuff each breast pocket with about 1/3 cup of the feta mixture; secure the pockets using wooden picks. Sprinkle the chicken evenly with salt and pepper.

- Heat oil in a large oven-safe skillet over medium-high heat. Arrange the stuffed breasts, top-sides down, in the pan; cook until golden, about 2 minutes. Carefully flip the chicken; transfer the pan to the oven. Bake until an instant-read thermometer inserted in the thickest portion of the chicken registers 165 degrees F, 20 to 25 minutes. Drizzle the chicken evenly with lemon juice. Remove the wooden picks from the chicken before serving.

Charred Shrimp & Pesto Buddha Bowls

Ingredients

- ⅓ cup prepared pesto
- 2 tablespoons balsamic vinegar
- 1 tablespoon extra-virgin olive oil
- ½ teaspoon salt
- ¼ teaspoon ground pepper

- 1 pound peeled and deveined large shrimp (16-20 count), patted dry
- 4 cups arugula
- 2 cups cooked quinoa
- 1 cup halved cherry tomatoes
- 1 avocado, diced

Directions

- Whisk pesto, vinegar, oil, salt and pepper in a large bowl. Remove 4 tablespoons of the mixture to a small bowl; set both bowls aside.
- Heat a large cast-iron skillet over medium-high heat. Add shrimp and cook, stirring, until just cooked through with a slight char, 4 to 5 minutes. Remove to a plate.
- Add arugula and quinoa to the large bowl with the vinaigrette and toss to coat. Divide the arugula mixture between 4 bowls. Top with tomatoes, avocado and shrimp. Drizzle each bowl with 1 tablespoon of the reserved pesto mixture.

Sheet-Pan Salmon with Sweet Potatoes & Broccoli

Ingredients

- 3 tablespoons low-fat mayonnaise
- 1 teaspoon chili powder
- 2 medium sweet potatoes, peeled and cut into 1-inch cubes
- 4 teaspoons olive oil, divided
- ½ teaspoon salt, divided
- ¼ teaspoon ground pepper, divided

- 4 cups broccoli florets (8 oz.; 1 medium crown)
- 1 ¼ pounds salmon fillet, cut into 4 portions
- 2 limes, 1 zested and juiced, 1 cut into wedges for serving
- ¼ cup crumbled feta or cotija cheese
- ½ cup chopped fresh cilantro

Directions

- Preheat oven to 425 degrees F. Line a large rimmed baking sheet with foil and coat with cooking spray.
- Combine mayonnaise and chili powder in a small bowl. Set aside.
- Toss sweet potatoes with 2 tsp. oil, 1/4 tsp. salt, and 1/8 tsp. pepper in a medium bowl. Spread on the prepared baking sheet. Roast for 15 minutes.
- Meanwhile, toss broccoli with the remaining 2 tsp. oil, 1/4 tsp. salt, and 1/8 tsp. pepper in the same bowl. Remove the baking sheet from oven. Stir the sweet potatoes and move them to the sides of the pan. Arrange salmon in the center of the pan and spread the broccoli on either side, among the sweet potatoes. Spread 2 Tbsp. of the mayonnaise mixture over the salmon. Bake until the sweet potatoes are tender and the salmon flakes easily with a fork, about 15 minutes.
- Meanwhile, add lime zest and lime juice to the remaining 1 Tbsp. mayonnaise; mix well.

- Divide the salmon among 4 plates and top with cheese and cilantro. Divide the sweet potatoes and broccoli among the plates and drizzle with the lime-mayonnaise sauce. Serve with lime wedges and any remaining sauce.

Mediterranean Ravioli with Artichokes & Olives

Ingredients

- 2 (8 ounce) packages frozen or refrigerated spinach-and-ricotta ravioli
- ½ cup oil-packed sun-dried tomatoes, drained (2 tablespoons oil reserved)
- 1 (10 ounce) package frozen quartered artichoke hearts, thawed
- 1 (15 ounce) can no-salt-added cannellini beans, rinsed
- ¼ cup Kalamata olives, sliced
- 3 tablespoons toasted pine nuts
- ¼ cup chopped fresh basil

Directions

- Bring a large pot of water to a boil. Cook ravioli according to package directions. Drain and toss with 1 tablespoon reserved oil; set aside.
- Heat the remaining 1 tablespoon oil in a large nonstick skillet over medium heat. Add artichokes and beans; sauté until heated through, 2 to 3 minutes.
- Fold in the cooked ravioli, sun-dried tomatoes, olives, pine nuts and basil.

Slow-Cooker Mediterranean Stew

Ingredients

- 2 (14 ounce) cans no-salt-added fire-roasted diced tomatoes
- 3 cups low-sodium vegetable broth
- 1 cup coarsely chopped onion
- ¾ cup chopped carrot
- 4 cloves garlic, minced
- 1 teaspoon dried oregano
- ¾ teaspoon salt
- ½ teaspoon crushed red pepper
- ¼ teaspoon ground pepper
- 1 (15 ounce) can no-salt-added chickpeas, rinsed, divided
- 1 bunch lacinato kale, stemmed and chopped (about 8 cups)
- 1 tablespoon lemon juice
- 3 tablespoons extra-virgin olive oil
- Fresh basil leaves, torn if large
- 6 lemon wedges (Optional)

Directions

- Combine tomatoes, broth, onion, carrot, garlic, oregano, salt, crushed red pepper and pepper in a 4-quart slow cooker. Cover and cook on Low for 6 hours.
- Measure 1/4 cup of the cooking liquid from the slow cooker into a small bowl. Add 2 tablespoons chickpeas; mash with a fork until smooth.
- Add the mashed chickpeas, kale, lemon juice and remaining whole chickpeas to the mixture in the slow cooker. Stir to

combine. Cover and cook on Low until the kale is tender, about 30 minutes.

- Ladle the stew evenly into 6 bowls; drizzle with oil. Garnish with basil. Serve with lemon wedges, if desired.

Greek Cauliflower Rice Bowls with Grilled Chicken

Ingredients

- 6 tablespoons plus 1 teaspoon extra-virgin olive oil, divided
- 4 cups cauliflower rice (see Tip)
- ⅓ cup chopped red onion
- ¾ teaspoon salt, divided
- ½ cup chopped fresh dill, divided
- 1 pound boneless, skinless chicken breasts
- ½ teaspoon ground pepper, divided
- 3 tablespoons lemon juice
- 1 teaspoon dried oregano
- 1 cup halved cherry tomatoes
- 1 cup chopped cucumber
- 2 tablespoons chopped Kalamata olives
- 2 tablespoons crumbled feta cheese
- 4 wedges Lemon wedges for serving

Directions

- Preheat grill to medium.
- Heat 2 tablespoons oil in a large skillet over medium-high heat. Add cauliflower, onion and 1/4 teaspoon salt. Cook, stirring occasionally, until the cauliflower is softened, about 5 minutes. Remove from heat and stir in 1/4 cup dill.

- Meanwhile, rub 1 teaspoon oil all over chicken. Sprinkle with 1/4 teaspoon salt and 1/4 teaspoon pepper. Grill, turning once, until an instant-read thermometer inserted into the thickest part of the breast reads 165 degrees F, about 15 minutes total. Slice crosswise.
- Meanwhile, whisk the remaining 4 tablespoons oil, lemon juice, oregano and the remaining 1/4 teaspoon each salt and pepper in a small bowl.
- Divide the cauliflower rice between 4 bowls. Top with the chicken, tomatoes, cucumber, olives and feta. Sprinkle with remaining 1/4 cup dill. Drizzle with the vinaigrette. Serve with lemon wedges, if desired.

Prosciutto Pizza with Corn & Arugula

Ingredients

- 1 pound pizza dough, preferably whole-wheat
- 2 tablespoons extra-virgin olive oil, divided
- 1 clove garlic, minced
- 1 cup part-skim shredded mozzarella cheese
- 1 cup fresh corn kernels
- 1 ounce very thinly sliced prosciutto, torn into 1-inch pieces
- 1 ½ cups arugula
- ½ cup torn fresh basil
- ¼ teaspoon ground pepper

Directions

- Preheat grill to medium-high. (Or to bake instead, see Tips.)

- Roll dough out on a lightly floured surface into a 12-inch oval. Transfer to a lightly floured large baking sheet. Combine 1 tablespoon oil and garlic in a small bowl. Bring the dough, the garlic oil, cheese, corn and prosciutto to the grill.

- Oil the grill rack (see Tips). Transfer the crust to the grill. Grill the dough until puffed and lightly browned, 1 to 2 minutes.

- Flip the crust over and spread the garlic oil on it. Top with the cheese, corn and prosciutto. Grill, covered, until the cheese is melted and the crust is lightly browned on the bottom, 2 to 3 minutes more. Return the pizza to the baking sheet.

- Top the pizza with arugula, basil and pepper. Drizzle with the remaining 1 tablespoon oil.

Cheesy Spinach-&-Artichoke Stuffed Spaghetti Squash

Ingredients

- 1 (2 1/2 to 3 pound) spaghetti squash, cut in half lengthwise and seeds removed
- 3 tablespoons water, divided
- 1 (5 ounce) package baby spinach
- 1 (10 ounce) package frozen artichoke hearts, thawed and chopped
- 4 ounces reduced-fat cream cheese, cubed and softened
- ½ cup grated Parmesan cheese, divided
- ¼ teaspoon salt
- ¼ teaspoon ground pepper
- Crushed red pepper & chopped fresh basil for garnish

Directions

- Place squash cut-side down in a microwave-safe dish; add 2 tablespoons water. Microwave, uncovered, on High until tender, 10 to 15 minutes. (Alternatively, place squash halves cut-side down on a rimmed baking sheet. Bake at 400 degrees F until tender, 40 to 50 minutes.)

- Meanwhile, combine spinach and the remaining 1 tablespoon water in a large skillet over medium heat. Cook, stirring occasionally, until wilted, 3 to 5 minutes. Drain and transfer to a large bowl.

- Position rack in upper third of oven; preheat broiler.

- Use a fork to scrape the squash from the shells into the bowl. Place the shells on a baking sheet. Stir artichoke hearts, cream cheese, 1/4 cup Parmesan, salt and pepper into the squash mixture. Divide it between the squash shells and top with the remaining 1/4 cup Parmesan. Broil until the cheese is golden brown, about 3 minutes. Sprinkle with crushed red pepper and basil, if desired.

Vegan Mediterranean Lentil Soup

Ingredients

- 2 tablespoons extra-virgin olive oil
- 1 ½ cups chopped yellow onions
- 1 cup chopped carrots
- 3 cloves garlic, minced
- 2 tablespoons no-salt-added tomato paste
- 4 cups reduced-sodium vegetable broth
- 1 cup water
- 1 (15 ounce) can no-salt-added cannellini beans, rinsed
- 1 cup mixed dry lentils (brown, green and black)
- ½ cup chopped sun-dried tomatoes in oil, drained
- ¾ teaspoon salt
- ½ teaspoon ground pepper
- 1 tablespoon chopped fresh dill, plus more for garnish
- 1 ½ teaspoons red-wine vinegar

Directions

- Heat oil in a large heavy pot over medium heat. Add onions and carrots; cook, stirring occasionally, until softened, 3 to 4 minutes. Add garlic and cook, stirring constantly, until fragrant, about 1 minute. Add tomato paste and cook, stirring constantly, until the mixture is evenly coated, about 1 minute.
- Stir in broth, water, cannellini beans, lentils, sun-dried tomatoes, salt and pepper. Bring to a boil over medium-high heat; reduce heat to medium-low to maintain a simmer. Cover and simmer until the lentils are tender, 30 to 40 minutes.
- Remove from heat and stir in dill and vinegar. Garnish with additional dill, if desired and serve.

EatingWell's Eggplant Parmesan

Ingredients

- Canola or olive oil cooking spray
- 2 large eggs
- 2 tablespoons water
- 1 cup panko breadcrumbs
- ¾ cup grated Parmesan cheese, divided
- 1 teaspoon Italian seasoning
- 2 medium eggplants (about 2 pounds total), cut crosswise into ¼-inch-thick slices
- ½ teaspoon salt
- ½ teaspoon ground pepper
- 1 (24 ounce) jar no-salt-added tomato sauce
- ¼ cup fresh basil leaves, torn, plus more for serving
- 2 cloves garlic, grated
- ½ teaspoon crushed red pepper
- 1 cup shredded part-skim mozzarella cheese, divided

Directions

- Position racks in middle and lower thirds of oven; preheat to 400°F. Coat 2 baking sheets and a 9-by-13-inch baking dish with cooking spray.

- Whisk eggs and water in a shallow bowl. Mix breadcrumbs, 1/4 cup Parmesan and Italian seasoning in another shallow dish. Dip eggplant in the egg mixture, then coat with the breadcrumb mixture, gently pressing to adhere.
- Arrange the eggplant in a single layer on the prepared baking sheets. Generously spray both sides of the eggplant with cooking spray. Bake, flipping the eggplant and switching the pans between racks halfway, until the eggplant is tender and lightly browned, about 30 minutes. Season with salt and pepper.
- Meanwhile, mix tomato sauce, basil, garlic and crushed red pepper in a medium bowl.
- Spread about 1/2 cup of the sauce in the prepared baking dish. Arrange half the eggplant slices over the sauce. Spoon 1 cup sauce over the eggplant and sprinkle with 1/4 cup Parmesan and 1/2 cup mozzarella. Top with the remaining eggplant, sauce and cheese.
- Bake until the sauce is bubbling and the top is golden, 20 to 30 minutes. Let cool for 5 minutes. Sprinkle with more basil before serving, if desired.

BBQ Shrimp with Garlicky Kale & Parmesan-Herb Couscous

Ingredients
- 1 cup low-sodium chicken broth
- ¼ teaspoon poultry seasoning
- ⅔ cup whole-wheat couscous
- ⅓ cup grated Parmesan cheese
- 1 tablespoon butter
- 3 tablespoons extra-virgin olive oil, divided
- 8 cups chopped kale
- ¼ cup water
- 1 large clove garlic, smashed
- ¼ teaspoon crushed red pepper
- ¼ teaspoon salt
- 1 pound peeled and deveined raw shrimp (26-30 per pound)
- ¼ cup barbecue sauce (see Tip)

Directions
- Combine broth and poultry seasoning in a medium saucepan over medium-high heat. Bring to a boil. Stir in couscous. Remove from heat, cover and let stand for 5 minutes. Fluff with a fork, then stir in Parmesan and butter. Cover to keep warm.
- Meanwhile, heat 1 tablespoon oil in large skillet over medium-high heat. Add kale and cook, stirring, until bright green, 1 to 2 minutes. Add water, cover and cook, stirring occasionally, until the kale is tender, about 3 minutes. Reduce heat to medium-low. Make a well in the center of the kale and add 1 tablespoon oil, garlic and crushed red pepper; cook, undisturbed, for 15 seconds, then stir the garlic oil into the kale and season with salt. Transfer to a bowl and cover to keep warm.
- Add the remaining 1 tablespoon oil and shrimp to the pan. Cook, stirring, until the

shrimp are pink and curled, about 2 minutes. Remove from heat and stir in barbecue sauce. Serve the shrimp with the kale and couscous.

Green Shakshuka with Spinach, Chard & Feta

Ingredients

- ⅓ cup extra-virgin olive oil
- 1 large onion, finely chopped
- 12 ounces chard, stemmed and chopped
- 12 ounces mature spinach, stemmed and chopped
- ½ cup dry white wine
- 1 small jalapeño or serrano pepper, thinly sliced
- 2 medium cloves garlic, very thinly sliced
- ¼ teaspoon kosher salt
- ¼ teaspoon ground pepper
- ½ cup low-sodium no-chicken or chicken broth
- 2 tablespoons unsalted butter
- 6 large eggs
- ½ cup crumbled feta or goat cheese

Directions

- Heat oil in a large skillet over medium heat. Add onion and cook, stirring often, until soft and translucent but not browned, 7 to 8 minutes. Add chard and spinach, a few handfuls at a time, and cook, stirring often, until wilted, about 5 minutes. Add wine, jalapeño (or serrano), garlic, salt and pepper; cook, stirring occasionally, until the wine is absorbed and the garlic softens, 2 to 4 minutes.

Add broth and butter; cook, stirring, until the butter is melted and some of the liquid is absorbed, 1 to 2 minutes.

- Crack eggs over the vegetables. Cover and cook over medium-low heat until the whites are set, 3 to 5 minutes. Remove from heat and sprinkle with cheese; cover and let stand for 2 minutes before serving.

One-Skillet Salmon with Fennel & Sun-Dried Tomato Couscous

Ingredients

- 1 lemon
- 1 ¼ pounds salmon (see Tip), skinned and cut into 4 portions
- ¼ teaspoon salt
- ¼ teaspoon ground pepper
- 4 tablespoons sun-dried tomato pesto, divided
- 2 tablespoons extra-virgin olive oil, divided
- 2 medium fennel bulbs, cut into 1/2-inch wedges; fronds reserved
- 1 cup Israeli couscous, preferably whole-wheat
- 3 scallions, sliced
- 1 ½ cups low-sodium chicken broth
- ¼ cup sliced green olives
- 2 tablespoons toasted pine nuts
- 2 cloves garlic, sliced

Directions

- Zest lemon and reserve the zest. Cut the lemon into 8 slices. Season salmon with salt and pepper and spread 1 1/2 teaspoons pesto on each piece.

- Heat 1 tablespoon oil in a large skillet over medium-high heat. Add half the fennel; cook until brown on the bottom, 2 to 3 minutes. Transfer to a plate. Reduce heat to medium and repeat with the remaining 1 tablespoon oil and fennel. Transfer to the plate. Add couscous and scallions to the pan; cook, stirring frequently, until the couscous is lightly toasted, 1 to 2 minutes. Stir in broth, olives, pine nuts, garlic, the reserved lemon zest and the remaining 2 tablespoons pesto.

- Nestle the fennel and salmon into the couscous. Top the salmon with the lemon slices. Reduce heat to medium-low, cover and cook until the salmon is cooked through and the couscous is tender, 10 to 14 minutes. Garnish with fennel fronds, if desired.

Chicken & Spinach Skillet Pasta with Lemon & Parmesan

Ingredients
- 8 ounces gluten-free penne pasta or whole-wheat penne pasta
- 2 tablespoons extra-virgin olive oil
- 1 pound boneless, skinless chicken breast or thighs, trimmed, if necessary, and cut into bite-size pieces
- ½ teaspoon salt
- ¼ teaspoon ground pepper
- 4 cloves garlic, minced

- ½ cup dry white wine
- Juice and zest of 1 lemon
- 10 cups chopped fresh spinach
- 4 tablespoons grated Parmesan cheese, divided

Directions
- Cook pasta according to package directions. Drain and set aside.

- Meanwhile, heat oil in a large high-sided skillet over medium-high heat. Add chicken, salt and pepper; cook, stirring occasionally, until just cooked through, 5 to 7 minutes. Add garlic and cook, stirring, until fragrant, about 1 minute. Stir in wine, lemon juice and zest; bring to a simmer.

- Remove from heat. Stir in spinach and the cooked pasta. Cover and let stand until the spinach is just wilted. Divide among 4 plates and top each serving with 1 tablespoon Parmesan.

Quinoa, Avocado & Chickpea Salad over Mixed Greens

Ingredients
- ⅔ cup water
- ⅓ cup quinoa
- ¼ teaspoon kosher salt or other coarse salt
- 1 clove garlic, crushed and peeled
- 2 teaspoons grated lemon zest
- 3 tablespoons lemon juice
- 3 tablespoons olive oil
- ¼ teaspoon ground pepper

- 1 cup rinsed no-salt-added canned chickpeas
- 1 medium carrot, shredded (1/2 cup)
- ½ avocado, diced
- 1 (5 ounce) package prewashed mixed greens, such as spring mix or baby kale-spinach blend (8 cups packed)

Directions

- Bring water to a boil in a small saucepan. Stir in quinoa. Reduce heat to low, cover, and simmer until all the liquid is absorbed, about 15 minutes. Use a fork to fluff and separate the grains; let cool for 5 minutes.
- Meanwhile, sprinkle salt over garlic on a cutting board. Mash the garlic with the side of a spoon until a paste forms. Scrape into a medium bowl. Whisk in lemon zest, lemon juice, oil, and pepper. Transfer 3 Tbsp. of the dressing to a small bowl and set aside.
- Add chickpeas, carrot, and avocado to the bowl with the remaining dressing; gently toss to combine. Let stand for 5 minutes to allow flavors to blend. Add the quinoa and gently toss to coat.
- Place greens in a large bowl and toss with the reserved 3 Tbsp. dressing. Divide the greens between 2 plates and top with the quinoa mixture.

Sheet-Pan Mediterranean Chicken, Brussels Sprouts & Gnocchi

Ingredients

- 4 tablespoons extra-virgin olive oil, divided
- 2 tablespoons chopped fresh oregano, divided
- 2 large cloves garlic, minced, divided
- ½ teaspoon ground pepper, divided
- ¼ teaspoon salt, divided
- 1 pound Brussels sprouts, trimmed and quartered
- 1 (16 ounce) package shelf-stable gnocchi
- 1 cup sliced red onion
- 4 boneless, skinless chicken thighs, trimmed
- 1 cup halved cherry tomatoes
- 1 tablespoon red-wine vinegar

Directions

- Preheat oven to 450 degrees F.
- Stir 2 tablespoons oil, 1 tablespoon oregano, half the garlic, 1/4 teaspoon pepper and 1/8 teaspoon salt together in a large bowl. Add Brussels sprouts, gnocchi and onion; toss to coat. Spread on a large rimmed baking sheet.
- Stir 1 tablespoon oil, the remaining 1 tablespoon oregano, the remaining garlic and the remaining 1/4 teaspoon pepper and 1/8 teaspoon salt in the large bowl. Add chicken and toss to coat. Nestle the chicken into the vegetable mixture. Roast for 10 minutes.
- Remove from the oven and add the tomatoes; stir to combine. Continue roasting until the Brussels sprouts are tender and the chicken is just cooked

through, about 10 minutes more. Stir vinegar and the remaining 1 tablespoon oil into the vegetable mixture.

Caprese Stuffed Portobello Mushrooms

Ingredients

- 3 tablespoons extra-virgin olive oil, divided
- 1 medium clove garlic, minced
- ½ teaspoon salt, divided
- ½ teaspoon ground pepper, divided
- 4 portobello mushrooms (about 14 ounces), stems and gills removed (see Tip)
- 1 cup halved cherry tomatoes
- ½ cup fresh mozzarella pearls, drained and patted dry
- ½ cup thinly sliced fresh basil
- 2 teaspoons best-quality balsamic vinegar

Directions

- Preheat oven to 400 degrees F.
- Combine 2 tablespoons oil, garlic, 1/4 teaspoon salt and 1/4 teaspoon pepper in a small bowl. Using a silicone brush, coat mushrooms all over with the oil mixture. Place on a large rimmed baking sheet and bake until the mushrooms are mostly soft, about 10 minutes.
- Meanwhile, stir tomatoes, mozzarella, basil and the remaining 1/4 teaspoon salt, 1/4 teaspoon pepper and 1 tablespoon oil together in a medium bowl. Once the mushrooms have

softened, remove from the oven and fill with the tomato mixture. Bake until the cheese is fully melted and the tomatoes have wilted, about 12 to 15 minutes more. Drizzle each mushroom with 1/2 teaspoon vinegar and serve.

Sweet & Spicy Roasted Salmon with Wild Rice Pilaf

Ingredients

- 5 skinless salmon fillets, fresh or frozen (1 1/4 lbs.)
- 2 tablespoons balsamic vinegar
- 1 tablespoon honey
- ¼ teaspoon salt
- ⅛ teaspoon ground pepper
- 1 cup chopped red and/or yellow bell pepper
- ½ to 1 small jalapeño pepper, seeded and finely chopped
- 2 scallions (green parts only), thinly sliced
- ¼ cup chopped fresh Italian parsley
- 2 2/3 cups Wild Rice Pilaf

Directions

- Thaw salmon, if frozen. Preheat oven to 425 degrees F. Line a 15-by-10-inch baking pan with parchment paper. Place the salmon in the prepared pan. Whisk vinegar and honey in a small bowl; drizzle half of the mixture over the salmon. Sprinkle with salt and pepper.
- Roast the salmon until the thickest part flakes easily, about 15 minutes. Drizzle with the remaining vinegar mixture.

- Coat a 10-inch nonstick skillet with cooking spray; heat over medium heat. Add bell pepper and jalapeño; cook, stirring frequently, just until tender, 3 to 5 minutes. Remove from heat. Stir in scallion greens.
- Top 4 of the salmon fillets with the pepper mixture and parsley. Serve with pilaf. (Refrigerate the remaining salmon for another use, see Note.)

Zucchini Lasagna Rolls with Smoked Mozzarella

Ingredients

- 2 large zucchini, trimmed
- 2 teaspoons extra-virgin olive oil
- ½ teaspoon ground pepper, divided
- ¼ teaspoon salt, divided
- 8 tablespoons shredded smoked mozzarella cheese, divided
- 3 tablespoons grated Parmesan cheese, divided
- 1 large egg, lightly beaten
- 1 ⅓ cups part-skim ricotta
- 1 (10 ounce) package frozen spinach, thawed and squeezed dry
- 1 clove garlic, minced
- ¾ cup low-sodium marinara sauce, divided
- 2 tablespoons chopped fresh basil

Directions

- Position racks in upper and lower thirds of oven; preheat to 425 degrees F. Coat 2 rimmed baking sheets with cooking spray.
- Slice zucchini lengthwise to get 24 total strips, about 1/8 inch thick each.
- Toss the zucchini, oil, 1/4 teaspoon pepper and 1/8 teaspoon salt in a large bowl. Arrange the zucchini in single layers on the prepared pans.
- Bake the zucchini, turning once, until tender, about 10 minutes total.
- Meanwhile, combine 2 tablespoons mozzarella and 1 tablespoon Parmesan in a small bowl. Set aside. Mix egg, ricotta, spinach, garlic and the remaining 6 tablespoons mozzarella, 2 tablespoons Parmesan, 1/4 teaspoon pepper and 1/8 teaspoon salt in a medium bowl.
- Spread 1/4 cup marinara in an 8-inch-square baking dish. Place 1 tablespoon of the ricotta mixture near the bottom of a strip of zucchini. Roll it up and place, seam-side down, in the baking dish. Repeat with the remaining zucchini and filling. Top the rolls with the remaining 1/2 cup marinara sauce and sprinkle with the reserved cheese mixture.
- Bake the zucchini rolls until bubbly and lightly browned on top, about 20 minutes. Let stand for 5 minutes. Sprinkle with basil before serving.

Herby Mediterranean Fish with Wilted

Ingredients

- 3 tablespoons olive oil, divided
- ½ large sweet onion, sliced
- 3 cups sliced cremini mushrooms

- 2 cloves garlic, sliced
- 4 cups chopped kale
- 1 medium tomato, diced
- 2 teaspoons Mediterranean Herb Mix (see Associated Recipes), divided
- 1 tablespoon lemon juice
- ½ teaspoon salt, divided
- ½ teaspoon ground pepper, divided
- 4 (4 ounce) cod, sole, or tilapia fillets
- Chopped fresh parsley, for garnish

Directions

- Heat 1 Tbsp. oil in a large saucepan over medium heat. Add onion; cook, stirring occasionally, until translucent, 3 to 4 minutes. Add mushrooms and garlic; cook, stirring occasionally, until the mushrooms release their liquid and begin to brown, 4 to 6 minutes. Add kale, tomato, and 1 tsp. herb mix. Cook, stirring occasionally, until the kale is wilted and the mushrooms are tender, 5 to 7 minutes. Stir in lemon juice and 1/4 tsp. each salt and pepper. Remove from heat, cover, and keep warm.

- Sprinkle fish with the remaining 1 tsp. herb mix and 1/4 tsp. each salt and pepper. Heat the remaining 2 Tbsp. oil in a large nonstick skillet over medium-high heat. Add the fish and cook until the flesh is opaque, 2 to 4 minutes per side, depending on thickness. Transfer the fish to 4 plates or a serving platter. Top and surround the fish with the vegetables; sprinkle with parsley, if desired.Greens & Mushrooms

Chicken with Tomato-Balsamic Pan Sauce

Ingredients

- 2 8-ounce boneless, skinless chicken breasts
- ½ teaspoon salt, divided
- ½ teaspoon ground pepper, divided
- ¼ cup white whole-wheat flour
- 3 tablespoons extra-virgin olive oil, divided
- ½ cup halved cherry tomatoes
- 2 tablespoons sliced shallot
- ¼ cup balsamic vinegar
- 1 cup low-sodium chicken broth
- 1 tablespoon minced garlic
- 1 tablespoon fennel seeds, toasted and lightly crushed
- 1 tablespoon butter

Directions

- Remove and reserve chicken tenders (if attached) for another use. Slice each breast in half horizontally to make 4 pieces total. Place on a cutting board and cover with a large piece of plastic wrap. Pound with the smooth side of a meat mallet or a heavy saucepan to an even thickness of about 1/4 inch. Sprinkle with 1/4 teaspoon each salt and pepper. Place flour in a shallow dish and dredge the cutlets to coat both sides, shaking off excess. (Discard remaining flour.)

- Heat 2 tablespoons oil in a large skillet over medium-high heat. Add 2 pieces of chicken and cook, turning once, until evenly browned and cooked through, 2 to 3 minutes per side. Transfer to a large serving plate and tent with foil to keep warm. Repeat with the remaining chicken.

- Add the remaining 1 tablespoon oil, tomatoes and shallot to the pan. Cook, stirring occasionally, until softened, 1 to 2 minutes. Add vinegar; bring to a boil. Cook, scraping up any browned bits from the bottom of the pan, until the vinegar is reduced by about half, about 45 seconds. Add broth, garlic, fennel seeds and the remaining 1/4 teaspoon salt and pepper. Cook, stirring, until the sauce is reduced by about half, 4 to 7 minutes. Remove from heat; stir in butter. Serve the sauce over the chicken.

Roasted Pistachio-Crusted Salmon with Broccoli

Ingredients

- 8 cups broccoli florets with 2-inch stalks attached
- 2 cloves garlic, sliced
- 3 tablespoons extra-virgin olive oil, divided
- ¾ teaspoon salt, divided
- ½ teaspoon ground pepper, divided
- ½ cup salted pistachios, coarsely chopped
- 2 tablespoons chopped fresh chives
- Zest of 1 medium lemon, plus wedges for serving

- 4 teaspoons mayonnaise
- 1 ¼ pounds salmon fillet, cut into 4 portions

Directions

- Preheat oven to 425 degrees F. Coat a large rimmed baking sheet with cooking spray.
- Combine broccoli, garlic, 2 tablespoons oil, 1/2 teaspoon salt and 1/4 teaspoon pepper on the prepared baking sheet. Roast for 5 minutes.
- Meanwhile, combine pistachios, chives, lemon zest, the remaining 1 tablespoon oil and 1/4 teaspoon each salt and pepper in a small bowl. Spread 1 teaspoon mayonnaise over each salmon portion and top with the pistachio mixture.
- Move the broccoli to one side of the baking sheet and place the salmon on the empty side. Roast until the salmon is opaque in the center and the broccoli is just tender, 8 to 15 minutes more, depending on thickness. Serve with lemon wedges, if desired.

Crispy Baked Ravioli with Red Pepper & Mushroom Bolognese

Ingredients

- Cooking spray
- 1 cup panko breadcrumbs, preferably whole-wheat
- ¼ cup finely grated Parmesan cheese, plus more for serving
- ½ teaspoon Italian seasoning

- 1 large egg
- 1 tablespoon water
- 1 pound fresh cheese ravioli (see Tip)
- 1 tablespoon extra-virgin olive oil
- 1 large red bell pepper, diced
- 2 cups chopped mushrooms
- ⅓ cup walnuts, finely chopped
- 2 cups low-sodium marinara sauce

Directions

- Preheat oven to 425 degrees F. Place a wire rack on a rimmed baking sheet and coat with cooking spray.
- Combine breadcrumbs, Parmesan and Italian seasoning in a shallow dish. Whisk egg and water in a separate shallow dish. Dip ravioli in the egg, letting excess drip off, then coat in the breadcrumb mixture, pressing to adhere. Place on the wire rack. Lightly coat the ravioli with cooking spray.
- Bake the ravioli until golden brown and crispy, about 15 minutes.
- Meanwhile, heat oil in a large saucepan over medium-high heat. Add bell pepper and mushrooms; cook, stirring, until softened, about 4 minutes. Add walnuts and cook, stirring, for 1 minute. Add marinara and cook until hot, about 2 minutes.
- Serve the ravioli with the sauce and more Parmesan, if desired.

Pan-Seared Halibut with Creamed Corn & Tomatoes

Ingredients

- 4 ears corn, husked
- 1 ½ cups whole milk
- 3 cloves garlic, divided
- 1 sprig fresh thyme
- 3 cups chopped tomatoes
- 3 tablespoons chopped fresh basil
- 2 tablespoons extra-virgin olive oil, divided
- ¾ teaspoon salt, divided
- 1 tablespoon butter
- ¼ cup chopped shallot
- 2 tablespoons all-purpose flour
- 2 tablespoons grated Parmesan cheese
- ½ teaspoon ground pepper, divided
- 1 ¼ pounds halibut, cut into 4 portions

Directions

- Put kernels from cobs and set aside. Cut or break the cobs in half and place in a large saucepan. Add milk, 2 garlic cloves and thyme. Cook over medium heat until starting to simmer around the edges. Remove from heat, cover and let steep for 10 minutes. Strain into a glass measuring cup or small bowl; discard the solids.
- Meanwhile, grate the remaining garlic clove into a medium bowl. Stir in tomatoes, basil, 1 tablespoon oil and 1/4 teaspoon salt. Set aside.
- Melt butter in the pan over medium heat. Add shallots and cook, stirring occasionally, until soft, about 1 minute. Add the reserved corn kernels and cook, stirring occasionally, until starting to soften, about 3 minutes. Sprinkle with

flour and cook for 30 seconds. While stirring, slowly add the milk. Adjust heat to maintain a simmer, cover and cook until thickened, about 5 minutes. Stir in Parmesan and 1/4 teaspoon each salt and pepper. Cover and set aside.

- Sprinkle halibut with the remaining 1/4 teaspoon each salt and pepper. Heat the remaining 1 tablespoon oil in a large nonstick skillet over medium-high heat. Add the halibut and cook, turning once, until lightly browned and just cooked through, 5 to 7 minutes total.

- Serve the halibut with the reserved creamed corn and tomatoes.

Greek Burgers with Herb-Feta Sauce

Ingredients

- 1 cup nonfat plain Greek yogurt
- ¼ cup crumbled feta cheese
- 3 tablespoons chopped fresh oregano, divided
- ¼ teaspoon lemon zest
- 2 teaspoons lemon juice
- ¾ teaspoon salt, divided
- 1 small red onion
- 1 pound ground lamb or ground beef
- ½ teaspoon ground pepper
- 2 whole-wheat pitas, halved, split and warmed
- 1 cup sliced cucumber
- 1 plum tomato, sliced

Directions

- Preheat grill to medium-high or preheat broiler to high.

- Mix yogurt, feta, 1 tablespoon oregano, lemon zest, lemon juice and 1/4 teaspoon salt in a small bowl.

- Cut 1/4-inch-thick slices of onion to make 1/4 cup. Finely chop more onion to make 1/4 cup. (Reserve any remaining onion for another use.) Mix the chopped onion and meat in a large bowl with the remaining 2 tablespoons oregano and 1/2 teaspoon each salt and pepper. Form into 4 oval patties, about 4 inches by 3 inches.

- Grill or broil the burgers, turning once, until an instant-read thermometer registers 160 degrees F, 4 to 6 minutes per side. Serve in pita halves, with the sauce, onion slices, cucumber and tomato.

Greek Roasted Fish with Vegetables

Ingredients

- 1 pound fingerling potatoes, halved lengthwise
- 2 tablespoons olive oil
- 5 garlic cloves, coarsely chopped
- ½ teaspoon sea salt
- ½ teaspoon freshly ground black pepper
- 4 5 to 6-ounce fresh or frozen skinless salmon fillets
- 2 medium red, yellow and/or orange sweet peppers, cut into rings
- 2 cups cherry tomatoes

- 1 ½ cups chopped fresh parsley (1 bunch)
- ¼ cup pitted kalamata olives, halved
- ¼ cup finely snipped fresh oregano or 1 Tbsp. dried oregano, crushed
- 1 lemon

Directions

- Preheat oven to 425 degrees F. Place potatoes in a large bowl. Drizzle with 1 Tbsp. of the oil and sprinkle with garlic and 1/8 tsp. of the salt and black pepper; toss to coat. Transfer to a 15x10-inch baking pan; cover with foil. Roast 30 minutes.
- Meanwhile, thaw salmon, if frozen. Combine, in the same bowl, sweet peppers, tomatoes, parsley, olives, oregano and 1/8 tsp. of the salt and black pepper. Drizzle with remaining 1 Tbsp. oil; toss to coat.
- Rinse salmon; pat dry. Sprinkle with remaining 1/4 tsp. salt and black pepper. Spoon sweet pepper mixture over potatoes and top with salmon. Roast, uncovered, 10 minutes more or just until salmon flakes.
- Remove zest from lemon. Squeeze juice from lemon over salmon and vegetables. Sprinkle with zest.

Easy Pea & Spinach Carbonara

Ingredients

- 1 ½ tablespoons extra-virgin olive oil
- ½ cup panko breadcrumbs, preferably whole-wheat

- 1 small clove garlic, minced
- 8 tablespoons grated Parmesan cheese, divided
- 3 tablespoons finely chopped fresh parsley
- 3 large egg yolks
- 1 large egg
- ½ teaspoon ground pepper
- ¼ teaspoon salt
- 1 (9 ounce) package fresh tagliatelle or linguine
- 8 cups baby spinach
- 1 cup peas (fresh or frozen)

Directions

- Put 10 cups of water in a large pot and bring to a boil over high heat.
- Meanwhile, heat oil in a large skillet over medium-high heat. Add breadcrumbs and garlic; cook, stirring frequently, until toasted, about 2 minutes. Transfer to a small bowl and stir in 2 tablespoons Parmesan and parsley. Set aside.
- Whisk the remaining 6 tablespoons Parmesan, egg yolks, egg, pepper and salt in a medium bowl.
- Cook pasta in the boiling water, stirring occasionally, for 1 minute. Add spinach and peas and cook until the pasta is tender, about 1 minute more. Reserve 1/4 cup of the cooking water. Drain and place in a large bowl.
- Slowly whisk the reserved cooking water into the egg mixture. Gradually add the mixture to the pasta, tossing with tongs

to combine. Serve topped with the reserved breadcrumb mixture.

MEDITERRANEAN SALAD RECIPES

Grilled Tofu with Mediterranean Salad

Total time: 45 minutes
Prep time: 30 minutes
Cook time: 15 minutes
Yield: 4 servings

Ingredients

- 1 tbsp. extra virgin olive oil
- ¼ cup lemon juice
- 2 tsp. dried oregano
- 3 cloves garlic, minced
- ½ tsp. sea salt
- Freshly ground pepper
- 14 ounces water-packed extra-firm tofu
- Mediterranean Chopped Salad
- 2 tbsp. extra virgin olive oil
- ¼ cup coarsely chopped Kalamata olives
- ¼ cup chopped scallions
- 1 cup diced seedless cucumber
- 2 medium tomatoes, diced
- ¼ cup chopped fresh parsley
- 1 tbsp. white-wine vinegar
- Freshly ground pepper
- ¼ tsp. sea salt

Directions

- Preheat your grill.
- In a small bowl, combine extra virgin olive oil, lemon juice, oregano, garlic, sea

salt and black pepper; reserve two tablespoons of the mixture for basting.

- Drain tofu and rinse; pat dry with paper towels. Cut tofu crosswise into 8 ½-inch thick slices and put in a glass dish.
- Add the lemon juice marinade and turn tofu to coat well.
- Marinate in the fridge for at least 30 minutes.
- In the meantime, prepare the salad.
- In a medium bowl, combine all the salad ingredients; toss gently to mix well.
- Set aside.
- Brush the grill rack with oil. Drain the marinated tofu and discard the marinade.
- Grill tofu over medium heat, for about 4 minutes per side, basting frequently with the remaining lemon juice marinade.
- Serve grilled tofu warm, topped with the salad.

Mediterranean Barley Salad

Total time: 1 hour 45 minutes
Prep time: 15 minutes
Cook time: 30 minutes
Chilling time: 1 hour
Yield: 6 servings

Ingredients

- 2 ½ cups water
- 1 cup barley
- 4 tbsp. extra virgin olive oil, divided
- 2 cloves garlic
- 7 sun-dried tomatoes
- 1 tbsp. balsamic vinegar
- ½ cup chopped black olives

- ½ cup finely chopped cilantro

Directions

- Mix water and barley in a saucepan; bring the mixture to a rolling boil over high heat.
- Lower heat to medium-low and simmer, covered, for about 30 minutes or until tender, but still a bit firm in the center.
- Drain and transfer to a large bowl; let the cooked barley cool to room temperature.
- In a blender, puree 2 tablespoons of extra virgin olive oil, garlic, sun-dried tomatoes, and balsamic vinegar until very smooth; pour over barley and fold in the remaining olive oil, olives, and cilantro.
- Refrigerate, covered, until chilled.
- Stir to mix well before serving.

Mediterranean Quinoa Salad

Total time: 35 minutes

Prep time: 15 minutes

Cook time: 20 minutes

Yield: 4 servings

Ingredients

- 1 clove garlic, smashed
- 2 cups water
- 2 cubes chicken bouillon
- 1 cup uncooked quinoa
- ½ cup chopped Kalamata olives
- 1 large red onion, diced
- 2 large chicken breasts (cooked), diced
- 1 large green bell pepper, diced
- ½ cup crumbled feta cheese
- ¼ cup chopped fresh chives

- ¼ cup chopped fresh parsley
- ½ tsp. sea salt
- ¼ cup extra virgin olive oil
- 1 tbsp. balsamic vinegar
- ⅔ cup fresh lemon juice

Directions

- Combine garlic clove, water, and bouillon cubes in a saucepan; bring the mixture to a gentle boil over medium-low heat.
- Stir in quinoa and simmer, covered, for about 20 minutes or until the water has been absorbed and quinoa is tender.
- Discard garlic clove and transfer the cooked quinoa to a large bowl.
- Stir in olives, onion, chicken, bell pepper, feta cheese, chives, parsley, sea salt, extra virgin olive oil, balsamic vinegar, and lemon juice.
- Serve warm or chilled.

Healthy Greek Salad

Total time: 15 minutes

Prep time: 15 minutes

Cook time: 0 minutes

Yield: 6 servings

Ingredients

- 1 small red onion, chopped
- 2 cucumbers, peeled and chopped
- 3 large ripe tomatoes, chopped
- 4 tsp. freshly squeezed lemon juice
- ¼ cup extra virgin olive oil
- 1 ½ tsp. dried oregano
- Sea salt
- Ground black pepper
- 6 pitted and sliced black Greek olives

- 1 cup crumbled feta cheese

Directions

- Combine onion, cucumber, and tomatoes in a shallow salad bowl; sprinkle with lemon juice, extra virgin olive, oregano, sea salt and black pepper.
- Sprinkle the olives and feta over the salad and serve immediately.

Almond, Mint and Kashi Salad

Total time: 1 hour 35 minutes

Prep time: 15 minutes

Cook time: 1 hour

Cooling time: 20 minutes

Yield: 4 servings

Ingredients

- 4 tbsp. extra virgin olive oil, divided, plus more for drizzling
- 1 small onion, finely chopped
- Sea salt, to taste
- Freshly ground black pepper, to taste
- 2 cups water
- 1 cup Kashi 7-Whole Grain Pilaf
- 2 bay leaves
- 3 tbsp. fresh lemon juice
- 5 tbsp. sliced natural almonds, divided
- 8 cherry tomatoes, quartered
- ¼ cup chopped parsley
- ¼ cup chopped fresh mint
- 4 large romaine leaves

Directions

- Heat 2 tablespoons of extra virgin olive oil in a large saucepan set over medium heat.
- Add onion, sea salt and pepper and cook, stirring occasionally, for about 5 minutes or until lightly browned and tender.
- Stir in 2 cups of water, Kashi, bay leaves, sea salt and pepper; bring the mixture to a rolling boil, lower heat to a simmer and cook, covered, for about 40 minutes or until Kashi is tender.
- Transfer to a large bowl and discard bay leaves, and then stir in the remaining extra virgin olive oil, and lemon juice.
- Let sit for at least 20 minutes or until cooled to room temperature.
- Adjust the seasoning if desired and add 4 tablespoons almonds, tomatoes, parsley, and mint; toss to mix well.
- Place one romaine leaf on each of the four plates and spoon the mixture into the center of the leaves; drizzle with extra virgin olive oil and sprinkle with the remaining almonds.

Chickpea Salad

Total time: 1 hour, 20 minutes

Prep time: 10 minutes

Cook time: 40 minutes

Standing time: 30 minutes

Yield: 6 servings

Ingredients

- 1 ½ cups dried chickpeas, soaked and liquid reserved
- 1 ¼ tsp. sea salt, divided
- 1 garlic clove, minced
- 2 tbsp. extra virgin olive oil
- 3 tbsp. sherry vinegar

- 16 crushed whole black peppercorns
- ¾ tsp. dried oregano
- 3 scallions, sliced into ½-inch pieces
- 2 carrots (4 ounces), cut into ½-inch dice
- 1 cup diced green bell pepper
- ½ English cucumber, peeled and diced
- 2 cups halved cherry tomatoes
- 2 tbsp. shredded fresh basil
- 3 tbsp. chopped fresh parsley

Directions

- Combine the chickpeas and soaking liquid in a large pot and season with ¾ teaspoons of sea salt.
- Bring the mixture to a gentle boil over medium heat. Lower heat to a simmer and cook, stirring occasionally, for about 40 minutes or until the chickpeas are tender; drain and transfer to a large bowl.
- In the meantime, mash together garlic and salt to form a paste; transfer to a separate bowl and stir in extra virgin olive oil, vinegar, peppercorns, and oregano to make the dressing.
- Pour the garlic dressing over the chickpeas and let stand for at least 30 minutes, stirring once.
- Toss in scallions, carrots, bell pepper, cucumber, tomatoes, basil, and parsley.
- Serve.

Italian Bread Salad

Total time: 2 hours 30 minutes

Prep time: 25 minutes, plus 2 hours Refrigerator time

Cook time: 5 minutes

Yield: 4 servings

Ingredients

- 3 tbsp. freshly squeezed lemon juice
- 2 tbsp. extra virgin olive oil
- Sea salt
- Freshly ground pepper
- 1 red onion, halved and sliced
- 1 bulb fennel, stalks removed and sliced
- 1 peeled English cucumber, sliced
- 1 ½ pounds diced tomatoes
- ⅓ cup pitted Kalamata olives, halved
- 4 slices whole-wheat country bread
- 1 garlic clove, peeled and halved
- 4 ounces shaved ricotta salata cheese
- ½ cup fresh basil leaves

Directions

- Whisk together lemon juice and extra virgin olive oil in a large bowl; season with sea salt and black pepper.
- Stir in onion, fennel, cucumber, tomatoes, and olives; toss to combine and refrigerate for about 2 hours.
- When ready, heat your broiler with the rack positioned 4 inches from heat and toast the bread on a baking sheet for about 2 minutes per side or until lightly browned.
- Transfer the toasted bread to a work surface and rub with the cut garlic and cut it into 2-inch pieces.
- Divide the bread among four shallow bowls and top with the tomato salad; sprinkle with cheese and basil to serve.

Bulgur Salad

Total time: 30 minutes

Prep time: 10 minutes

Cook time: 20 minutes

Yield: 4 servings

Ingredients

- 1 tbsp. unsalted butter
- 2 tbsp. extra virgin olive oil, divided
- 2 cups bulgur
- 4 cups water
- ¼ tsp. sea salt
- 1 medium cucumber, deseeded and chopped
- ¼ cup dill, chopped
- 1 handful black olives, pitted and chopped
- 2 tsp. red wine vinegar

Directions

- Place a saucepan over medium heat and add 1 tbsp. of butter and 1 tbsp. of olive oil.
- Toast the bulgur in the oil until it turns golden brown and starts to crackle.
- Add 4 cups of water to the saucepan and season with the salt.
- Cover the saucepan and simmer until all the water gets absorbed for about 20 minutes.
- In a mixing bowl, combine the chopped cucumber with dill, olives, red wine vinegar and the remaining olive oil.
- Serve this over the bulgur.

Greek Salad

Total time: 20 minutes

Prep time: 20 minutes

Cook time: 0 minutes

Yield: 4 servings

Ingredients

- Juice of 1 lemon
- 6 tbsp. extra virgin olive oil
- Black pepper to taste, ground
- 1 tsp. oregano, dried
- 1 head romaine lettuce, washed, dried and chopped
- 1 red bell pepper, chopped
- 1 green bell pepper, chopped
- 1 cucumber, sliced
- 2 tomatoes, chopped
- 1 cup feta cheese, crumbled
- 1 red onion, thinly sliced
- 1 can black olives, pitted

Directions

- Whisk together the lemon juice, olive oil, pepper and oregano in a small bowl.
- In a large bowl, combine the lettuce, bell peppers, cucumber, tomatoes, cheese and onion.
- Pour the salad dressing into this bowl and toss until evenly coated with the dressing, then serve.

Potato Salad

Total time: 24 minutes

Prep time: 10 minutes

Cook time: 14 minutes

Yield: 4 servings

Ingredients

- 5 medium potatoes, peeled and diced
- Coarse salt, to taste
- ¼ onion
- 3 tbsp. yellow mustard
- 2 cups mayonnaise
- 1 tsp. paprika, sweet
- 1 tsp. Tabasco
- 2 scallions, thinly sliced

Directions

- Pour some water in a saucepan and place over medium heat.
- Add the potatoes, season with coarse salt and boil for around 10 minutes until tender.
- Drain the water and return the saucepan to the heat to dry them out.
- Let the potatoes cool to room temperature.
- Grate the onion in a mixing bowl, add mustard, mayo, paprika and the hot sauce and mix well.
- Add the potatoes to the bowl and toss until evenly coated.
- Divide among four bowls and top with the sliced scallions.

Mediterranean Green Salad

Total time: 25 minutes

Prep time: 15 minutes

Cook time: 10 minutes

Yield: 4 servings

Ingredients

- ½ loaf rustic sourdough bread
- ¼ tsp. paprika
- 2 tbsp. manchego, finely grated
- 7 tbsp. extra virgin olive oil, divided
- 1 ½ tbsp. sherry vinegar
- ½ tsp. sea salt
- 1 tsp. freshly ground black pepper
- 1 tsp. Dijon mustard
- 5 cups mixed baby greens
- ¾ cup green olives, pitted and halved
- 12 thin slices of Serrano ham, roughly chopped

Directions

- Cut the bread into bite-sized cubes and set aside.
- Preheat oven to 400°F.
- In a mixing bowl, combine paprika, manchego and 6 tbsps. of olive oil.
- Add the bread cubes and toss them until they are evenly coated with the flavored oil.
- Arrange the bread on a baking sheet and bake for about 8 minutes until golden brown and let the bread cool.
- In a separate bowl, combine the vinegar, salt, pepper, mustard and the remaining olive oil.
- Add this mixture to a larger bowl containing the greens until they are lightly coated with the vinaigrette.
- Add all the other ingredients and the croutons and toss well.
- Serve the salad on four plates.

Chickpea Salad with Yogurt Dressing

Total time: 30 minutes

Prep time: 30 minutes

Cook time: 0 minutes

Yield: 4 servings

Ingredients

Dressing

- 1 tbsp. freshly squeezed lemon juice
- 1 cup plain nonfat Greek yogurt
- ¼ tsp. cayenne pepper
- 1½ tsp. curry powder

Salad

- 2 15-oz. cans chickpeas, rinsed and drained
- 1 cup diced red apple
- ½ cup diced celery
- ¼ cup chopped walnuts
- ¼ cup thinly sliced green onions
- ⅓ cup raisins
- ½ cup chopped fresh parsley
- 2 lemon wedges

Directions

- Make dressing: In a small bowl, whisk together lemon juice, yogurt, cayenne, and curry powder until well combined.
- Make salad: In a large bowl, toss together chickpeas, apple, celery, walnuts, green onions, raisins, and parsley.
- Gently fold in the dressing and season with sea salt and pepper.
- Serve garnished with lemon wedges.

Warm Lentil Salad

Total time: 20 minutes

Prep time: 10 minutes

Cook time: 10 minutes

Yield: 4 servings

Ingredients

- 3 tbsp. extra virgin olive oil
- 1 ½ cups thinly sliced leeks
- 2 tsp. whole-grain mustard
- 2 tbsp. sherry vinegar
- 2 cups cooked lentils
- 1 ½ cups red grapes, halved
- ¼ cup chopped roasted pistachios
- ¼ cup crumbled feta
- 3 tbsp. finely chopped parsley
- 3 tbsp. finely chopped mint

Directions

- In a skillet, heat extra virgin olive oil over medium heat; add leeks and sauté, stirring, for about 9 minutes or until translucent and tender.
- Remove the pan from heat and stir in mustard and sherry vinegar.
- In a large bowl, combine the leek mixture, lentils, grapes, pistachios, mint, parsley, sea salt, and pepper.
- Top with feta and enjoy!

TUNA SALAD WITH TOASTED PINE NUTS

Tarragon is an herb from southern France that has a delicate anise flavor. Use it in fish and chicken dishes.

Serves 4

- 1 (5-ounce) can tuna, packed in olive oil, drained and flaked 1 medium shallot, diced
- 3 tablespoons chopped fresh chives
- 1 tablespoon chopped fresh tarragon
- 1 stalk celery, trimmed and finely diced 2–3 tablespoons mayonnaise
- 1 teaspoon Dijon mustard
- 1/4 teaspoon salt 1/8 teaspoon pepper
- 1/4 cup toasted pine nuts

Directions

- In a medium bowl, toss the tuna, shallot, chives, tarragon, and celery.
- In a small bowl, combine the mayonnaise, mustard, salt, and pepper. Stir the mayonnaise mixture into the tuna mixture. Stir in the pine nuts. Serve cool or at room temperature.

WATERMELON AND FETA SALAD

Serves 4

- 4 1/4 cups cubed (3/4-inch)
- watermelon, divided
- 1/3 cup sliced red onions
- 1/3 cup purslane leaves
- 1 1/2 cups cubed (3/4-inch) feta
- 1/4 cup fresh mint leaves
- 1 teaspoon honey
- 1 tablespoon fresh lemon juice
- 1/4 cup extra-virgin olive oil

Directions

- In a large bowl, combine 4 cups of the watermelon, onions, purslane, and feta.

- Place the remaining watermelon, mint, honey, lemon juice, and oil in a food processor. Process until the dressing is well incorporated.
- Pour the dressing over the salad and toss gently with your fingers to combine. Serve cool or at room temperature.

BULGUR SALAD WITH NUTS, HONEY, CHEESE, AND POMEGRANATE

Serves 4

- 1 cup coarse (#3) bulgur wheat
- 1 teaspoon salt
- 1/2 cup extra-virgin olive oil
- 1/4 cup chopped toasted almonds (see Toasting Nuts sidebar)
- 1/4 cup chopped toasted walnuts
- 1/4 teaspoon ground allspice
- 1/4 cup pomegranate molasses
- 2 teaspoons red wine vinegar
- 2 teaspoons honey
- 2 scallions, ends trimmed, thinly sliced
- 1 1/2 cups baby arugula, washed and dried
- 1/4 cup chopped fresh mint
- 1 cup crumbled goat cheese
- 1/4 teaspoon pepper

Directions

- Fill a medium pot two-thirds with water and set it over medium-high heat. Bring the water to a boil. Add bulgur and salt. Boil for 6 minutes. Strain the bulgur.

- While the bulgur is still warm, add oil, nuts, allspice, molasses, vinegar, and honey. Mix well.
- Add the scallions, arugula, mint, cheese, and pepper. Toss to combine. Adjust seasoning with more salt and pepper, if necessary.
- Serve at room temperature.

CREAMY COLESLAW

Serves 6

- 1 1/2 teaspoons salt
- 1 tablespoon sugar
- 1/4 cup red wine vinegar
- 1/2 large head cabbage, stalk removed and thinly sliced
- 1 large peeled carrot, grated
- 2 scallions, ends trimmed and thinly sliced
- 2 cloves garlic, peeled and minced
- 1/2 cup extra-virgin olive oil
- 1/4 cup mayonnaise
- 1/2 cup strained Greek yogurt Salt and pepper to season (optional)

Directions

- In a large bowl, whisk together sugar, salt, and vinegar. Add the cabbage, carrot, scallions, and garlic. Toss to combine. Let the vegetables sit for 5 minutes.
- To the vegetables, add the oil, mayonnaise, and yogurt. Stir to combine and coat the vegetables in the creamy dressing.

- Adjust the seasoning with more salt and pepper, if necessary. Serve the coleslaw cool or at room temperature.

ARUGULA, PEAR, AND GOAT CHEESE SALAD

Arugula is a peppery salad green that is sometimes called "rocket" in grocery stores.

Serves 4

- 2 medium pears, cored and cut into wedges
- 2 tablespoons fresh lemon juice, divided
- 1 tablespoon balsamic vinegar
- 1/3 cup extra-virgin olive oil
- 1/4 cup chopped fresh chives
- 1/2 teaspoon salt
- 1/8 teaspoon pepper
- 3 cups arugula, rinsed and dried
- 1/2 cup chopped unsalted pistachios
- 1/2 cup crumbled goat cheese

Directions

- In a small bowl, toss the pears with 1 tablespoon of the lemon juice. In a large bowl, whisk remaining lemon juice, vinegar, oil, chives, salt, and pepper.
- Toss the arugula in the dressing and plate it on a serving platter. Arrange the pears over the arugula and sprinkle the top with pistachios and cheese. Drizzle any remaining dressing over the salad and serve.

GREEK VILLAGE SALAD

Serves 4

- 4 medium-size ripe tomatoes, cut into wedges
- 1/2 English cucumber, halved and sliced into 1/2-inch slices
- 1 medium cubanelle (green) pepper, stemmed, seeded, halved, and cut into slices
- 1 small red onion, peeled, halved, and thinly sliced
- 1/8 teaspoon salt 1/3 cup extra-virgin olive oil
- 1 1/2 cups cubed feta cheese
- 1 teaspoon dried oregano
- 8 kalamata olives

Directions

- On a serving plate, arrange tomatoes and cucumbers. Next add peppers and onions. Season vegetables with salt.
- Drizzle oil over the vegetables. Top with feta and sprinkle with oregano.
- Finally, top the salad with the olives and serve at room temperature.

STRAWBERRY AND FETA SALAD WITH BALSAMIC DRESSING

Serves 4

- 1 teaspoon Dijon mustard
- 3 tablespoons balsamic vinegar
- 1 clove garlic, peeled and minced
- 3/4 cup extra-virgin olive oil
- 1/2 teaspoon salt
- 1/8 teaspoon pepper
- 4 cups salad greens, rinsed and dried

- 1 pint ripe strawberries, hulled and halved
- 1 1/2 cups crumbled feta cheese

Directions

- In a small bowl, whisk the mustard, vinegar, garlic, oil, salt, and pepper to make the dressing.
- In a large bowl, combine the salad greens and the dressing. Plate the salad on a serving platter and top with the strawberries and feta.
- Drizzle any remaining dressing over the salad and serve.

CREAMY CAESAR SALAD

This recipe makes more dressing than you'll need for this salad. Add as much or as little dressing as you prefer. Leftover dressing can be stored in the refrigerator for up to one week.
Serves 6

- 2 cloves garlic, peeled and chopped
- 3 egg yolks
- 1 tablespoon Dijon mustard
- 3 tablespoons Worcestershire sauce
- 1 tablespoon anchovy paste or 2 anchovy fillets
- 1/2 cup grated Parmesan cheese, divided 2 tablespoons fresh lemon juice, divided
- 1/2 teaspoon salt 1 teaspoon pepper
- 1 tablespoon water
- 1 cup light olive oil
- 1 head romaine lettuce, washed, dried, and chopped 1/2 cup chopped cooked bacon 1 cup croutons

Directions

- Place the garlic, egg yolks, mustard, Worcestershire sauce, anchovy paste, 1/4 cup Parmesan cheese, 1 tablespoon lemon juice, salt, pepper, and water into the food processor. Process until the dressing is combined and thick. With the processor running, slowly add the oil until it is well incorporated. Taste the dressing and adjust the seasoning with more salt and pepper, if necessary.

- In a large bowl, combine the lettuce and the remaining lemon juice. Add just enough dressing to coat the lettuce (add more if you want to make it creamier). Toss in the bacon and croutons. Top the salad with the remaining Parmesan. Serve with extra dressing.

POLITIKI CABBAGE SALAD

Serves 4

- 1 teaspoon sugar
- 1 teaspoon salt
- 1/4 cup red wine vinegar
- 4 cups shredded white cabbage
- 1/2 cup grated peeled carrot
- 1/2 cup thinly sliced red pepper
- 1/4 cup celery, diced
- 1/4 cup extra-virgin olive oil
- 1/8 teaspoon red pepper flakes Salt and pepper to season (optional)

Directions

- In a large bowl, whisk sugar, salt, and vinegar. Add the cabbage, carrot, pepper, and celery. Toss to combine. Let

the vegetables sit for 15–20 minutes. The vegetables will begin to release liquid.

- Using your hands, squeeze out any excess liquid from the vegetables and place them in a separate large bowl.

- To the vegetables, add the oil and red pepper flakes. Toss to coat the vegetables in the oil. Adjust the seasoning with more salt and pepper, if necessary. Serve the salad cool or at room temperature.

ARUGULA SALAD WITH FIGS AND SHAVED CHEESE

Serves 6

- 1 tablespoon honey
- 1 teaspoon Dijon mustard
- 3 tablespoons balsamic vinegar
- 1 small clove garlic, peeled and minced
- 1 teaspoon salt
- 1/2 teaspoon pepper
- 2/3 cup extra-virgin olive oil
- 5 cups arugula leaves, rinsed and dried
- 12 fresh (ripe) figs, stemmed and quartered
- 1 cup walnuts, roughly chopped
- 1/4 cup shaved Graviera or Gruyère cheese

Directions

- In a large bowl, whisk honey, mustard, vinegar, garlic, salt, and pepper. Slowly whisk in the oil until well incorporated.

- Add the arugula and figs. Toss the salad to combine the ingredients and to coat them in the dressing.
- Sprinkle the salad with walnuts and cheese, and serve.

SPINACH SALAD WITH APPLES AND MINT

Use any variety of apples you like for this salad. Always include at least one tart apple.

Serves 4

- 1/3 cup extra-virgin olive oil 10 fresh mint leaves, chopped
- 1 large orange, peeled and segmented, juice reserved
- 1 large grapefruit, peeled and segmented, juice reserved
- 1 tablespoon fresh lime juice
- 3/4 teaspoon salt
- 1/4 teaspoon pepper
- 1 large red apple, cored and cut into thin slices
- 1 large green apple, cored and cut into thin slices
- 1/3 cup finely chopped red onion
- 1 stalk celery, trimmed and chopped
- 4 cups baby spinach, washed and dried

Directions

- Put the oil and mint into a food processor. Process until well incorporated. Set aside and let the mint infuse the oil.
- In a large bowl, whisk together reserved orange juice, grapefruit juice, lime juice, salt, pepper, and olive oil–mint infusion.

Add the apple slices, onion, and celery. Toss the salad to coat in the dressing.

- Add the spinach and toss again to combine with the salad and dressing. Top the salad with orange and grapefruit segments, and serve.

TOMATO SALAD WITH FRIED FETA

Keep your fried cheese warm in a preheated 280°F oven until you are ready to serve.

Serves 4

- 1 large egg
- 1 teaspoon whole milk
- 1/4 cup all-purpose flour 1 1/2 cups feta cheese, cut into 1/2-inch cubes
- 1 tablespoon fresh lemon juice
- 1 2/3 cups extra-virgin olive oil, divided 1 teaspoon Dijon mustard
- 1 tablespoon balsamic vinegar
- 1 teaspoon honey
- 2 teaspoons dried oregano
- 1 teaspoon salt
- 1/4 teaspoon pepper 2 medium-size ripe tomatoes, sliced into 1/2-inch slices 4 cups salad greens, rinsed and dried
- 1 small red onion, thinly sliced
- 1/2 cup kalamata olives

Directions

- In a small bowl, beat the egg and milk. Put the flour into another small bowl. Dip the feta cubes in the egg mixture and then dredge them in the flour. Shake off any excess flour. Refrigerate the dredged feta for at least 30 minutes.
- Into a small jar with a lid, put the lemon juice, 2/3 cup oil, mustard, vinegar,

honey, oregano, salt, and pepper. Close the jar and shake vigorously until the dressing is well incorporated.

- Add the remaining oil to a medium nonstick frying pan and heat on medium for 1 minute. Add the feta (in batches) and fry until the cubes are lightly golden on all sides (20–30 seconds per side). Place the feta on a tray lined with paper towels to absorb any excess oil.

- In a large bowl, place the tomatoes, greens, onions, and olives. Shake the dressing and then add it to the salad. Toss to combine the ingredients.

POTATO SALAD

Serves 6

- 6 large Yukon gold potatoes, skins on
- 1 1/2 teaspoons salt
- 1/2 teaspoon pepper
- 1/2 cup extra-virgin olive oil
- 1/4 cup Dijon mustard
- 2 tablespoons capers, drained and chopped
- 1/4 cup red wine vinegar
- 2 tablespoons chopped fresh parsley
- 3 scallions, ends trimmed and finely chopped
- 1/2 cup chopped fresh dill
- 1 tablespoon fresh lemon juice

Directions

- Place a large pot of water over medium-high heat. Add the potatoes and bring the water to a boil. Cook for 30 minutes. Let potatoes cool for 10 minutes, and

then peel them. Cut the potatoes into chunks.

- In a large bowl, whisk the remaining ingredients until they are well incorporated.

- Add the potatoes to the dressing and toss to coat. Serve the salad warm or at room temperature.

WARM MUSHROOM SALAD

This is a wonderful, hearty winter salad.

Serves 4

- 2/3 cup extra-virgin olive oil, divided 2 cups sliced cremini mushrooms
- 2 cups sliced king mushrooms
- 6 cloves garlic, peeled and smashed
- 2 bay leaves
- 1 teaspoon chopped fresh rosemary
- 1 teaspoon fresh thyme leaves
- 1 teaspoon salt, divided
- 1/2 teaspoon pepper, divided 1 teaspoon Dijon mustard
- 2 tablespoons balsamic vinegar
- 1 tablespoon fresh lemon juice
- 4 cups salad greens, washed and dried
- 1/4 cup pumpkin seeds
- 1/2 cup crumbled goat cheese
- 1/4 cup crispy fried onions (see Crispy Fried Onions sidebar)

Directions

- Heat 1/3 cup oil in a large cast-iron pan over medium-low heat for 30 seconds. Add the mushrooms, garlic, bay leaves, rosemary, thyme, 1/2 teaspoon salt, and 1/4 teaspoon pepper. Stirring occasionally, cook the mushrooms for 20 minutes, then remove bay leaves.

- In a small jar with a lid, place the remaining oil, mustard, vinegar, lemon juice, and remaining salt and pepper. Close the jar and shake it vigorously until the dressing is well incorporated.
- In a large bowl, add the greens and dressing and toss them to combine. Divide and plate the greens, and then top them with the warm mushrooms. Sprinkle the salad with the pumpkin seeds, cheese, and crispy fried onions. Drizzle the remaining dressing over the salads. Serve them warm or at room temperature.

SUN-DRIED TOMATO VINAIGRETTE

Use this dressing with spinach or peppery salad greens.

Serves 4

- 1⁄3 cup sun-dried tomatoes, packed in olive oil, rinsed and finely chopped 2 tablespoons balsamic vinegar
- 1 teaspoon garlic powder
- 1 teaspoon dried oregano
- 1⁄4 teaspoon pepper
- 1⁄2 teaspoon salt
- 1⁄3 cup extra-virgin olive oil

Directions

- In a small bowl, whisk all the ingredients until they are well incorporated.
- Keep the dressing refrigerated until it is needed.

CREAMY FETA DRESSING

Spoon this dressing over olive oil fries, a baked potato, or a vegetable tray.

Serves 4

- 1⁄3 cup crumbled feta cheese
- 2 teaspoons water
- 3⁄4 cup plain yogurt
- 2 tablespoons mayonnaise
- 2 tablespoons evaporated milk
- 1 teaspoon dried oregano
- 1 clove garlic, peeled and minced
- 2 tablespoons chopped fresh chives
- 1⁄8 teaspoon pepper

Directions

- Place the feta and water in a medium bowl. Using a fork, mash the feta into a paste.
- Add the remaining ingredients and mix them until they are well incorporated. Keep the dressing refrigerated until it is needed.

KALAMATA OLIVE DRESSING

Serves 4

- 1⁄4 cup chopped red onions
- 1 clove garlic, peeled and smashed
- 1⁄2 cup pitted kalamata olives
- 2 sun-dried tomatoes, packed in olive oil, rinsed and chopped
- 1⁄2 teaspoon dried oregano
- 2 tablespoons red wine vinegar
- 1 tablespoon balsamic vinegar
- 1 teaspoon Dijon mustard
- 1⁄2 teaspoon pepper

- 2/3 cup extra-virgin olive oil

Directions

- Add all the ingredients to a food processor, and process until they are well incorporated.
- Refrigerate the dressing until it is needed.

CUCUMBER AND DILL DRESSING

This dressing pairs wonderfully with salad greens, ripe tomatoes, and some peppery radish slices.

Serves 4

- 1/2 medium English cucumber, grated
- 3/4 teaspoon salt, divided
- 1/2 cup strained Greek yogurt
- 1/4 cup whole milk
- 2 tablespoons mayonnaise
- 2 teaspoons fresh lemon juice
- 1 scallion (white part only), ends trimmed and thinly sliced
- 1 clove garlic, peeled and minced
- 2 tablespoons chopped fresh dill
- 1/4 teaspoon pepper

Directions

- Place cucumber and 1/4 teaspoon salt in a fine-mesh strainer over a medium bowl. Strain for 30 minutes. Squeeze any remaining water from the cucumber.
- Combine the cucumber and remaining ingredients in a medium bowl. Stir well to incorporate the ingredients.

- Adjust the seasoning if necessary. Refrigerate the dressing in a tight jar for up to 1 week.

GRILLED EGGPLANT SALAD

Serves 4

- 1 large eggplant
- 2 tablespoons salt, plus more to taste
- 2 or 3 tomatoes
- Small bunch of parsley, finely chopped
- 2 cloves garlic, pressed or very finely diced Pepper to taste
- 1 tablespoon dried oregano
- 1/4 cup extra-virgin olive oil

Directions

- Slice eggplant into discs along length—not too thin and not too thick, about 1/4 inch thickness is ideal. Fill a large mixing bowl or pot with water, add 2 tablespoons of salt, and mix well; place eggplant discs in salt bath and set a plate over the top to weigh them down. Soak for 20–30 minutes. Mix periodically to ensure salty water soaks them completely.
- Dice tomatoes; place in bowl. Add parsley, garlic, salt, pepper, oregano, and 2–3 tablespoons olive oil; mix well and set aside.
- Light a grill and set on high temperature. When grilling surface is ready, spray or wipe with vegetable oil.
- Using your hands and working quickly over the grill, brush (or spray) downward-facing side of each slice of eggplant with

a little olive oil; place across grill, starting from the top left rear section and filling the entire surface in rows. Once all the eggplant discs are on the grill, give the upward-facing sides a brush (or spray) of olive oil. Grill until visibly softened around the edges and centers, approximately 6–8 minutes. Allow each side a few minutes to cook through and absorb oil, but watch them carefully.

- Brush with olive oil again; turn over. Grill another few minutes; give final brushing of oil. Leave on grill another minute or so; remove onto platter or dish.

- Arrange several eggplant discs on a serving plate, top with chopped tomato mixture, sprinkle with oregano, and serve with crusty bread.

LAHANOSALATA (CABBAGE SALAD)

Serves 4

- 1/3 of a white cabbage
- 2 large carrots
- 1/2 cup Greek-style strained yogurt
- 1/4 cup extra-virgin olive oil
- 2 tablespoons fresh lemon juice (or vinegar)
- 1/2 teaspoon dried oregano
- 1 tablespoon chopped fresh dill Salt and pepper to taste

Directions

- Wash cabbage well; peel carrots. Shred cabbage finely with a sharp knife. Shred carrots into ribbons using a mandoline or the large holes on a grater; add to shredded cabbage.

- Toss shredded cabbage and carrots well.

- In a food processor/blender, add yogurt, olive oil, lemon juice, oregano, dill, salt, and pepper; blend together until smooth and creamy.

- Pour the dressing over the top of individual servings or mix well into the entire salad before serving. Garnish with chopped dill and a kalamata olive or two.

TARAMOSALATA/TARAMA (FISH ROE SALAD)

Serves 6–8

- 1/2 loaf two-day-old white bread
- 1/2 cup carp roe 1 large onion, grated Juice of 2 lemons
- 2 cups extra-virgin olive oil
- Cucumber slices, for garnish
- Tomato slices, for garnish
- Olives, for garnish

Directions

- Remove the outside crust and soak the inner bread in water; squeeze well to drain and set aside.

- Place fish roe in a food processor/blender; mix a minute or so to break down eggs.

- Add grated onion to the processor; continue mixing.

- Add moistened bread in stages to the processor/blender; mix well.

- Slowly add lemon juice and olive oil while constantly mixing. Note: When adding olive oil and lemon juice, add in a slow and alternate fashion by first adding some lemon juice then some olive oil and so on, until both are incorporated into the tarama.

- Refrigerate before serving to firm up the tarama. Garnish with cucumber, tomato slices, and/or olive(s); serve with warm pita bread.

GRILLED HALLOUMI SALAD

Serves 4

- 10–12 kalamata olives, pitted and finely chopped or ground to a pulp
- 1/4 cup extra-virgin olive oil 2 tablespoons balsamic vinegar
- 1 tablespoon dried oregano
- 1 medium carrot, shredded
- 1/4 of a small green cabbage, shredded
- 1 large tomato
- 1 bunch fresh rocket greens (arugula), finely cut
- 1 head romaine lettuce, finely cut
- 2 stalks fresh green onion, finely sliced (green stalk included)
- 1/2 pound halloumi cheese, thick sliced

Directions

- Prepare the dressing by pitting and grinding or finely chopping olives; combine pulp with olive oil, vinegar, and oregano. Mix well; set aside.
- Wash all the vegetables well. Peel carrot; use a mandoline to finely shred cabbage and carrot into a large salad bowl. Chop tomato into sections; add to the bowl.

Finely cut rocket and lettuce; add to the bowl. Finely slice green onions; add to salad.

- Fire up a grill; grill the halloumi until it noticeably starts to soften and grill marks appear. Make sure to flip the cheese so both sides are scored with grill marks. When the cheese is done, remove from heat and immediately cut into cubes; add to salad. Pour dressing over the salad; mix well. Serve immediately.

GRILLED BANANA PEPPER SALAD

If you don't like hot peppers, make sure to choose sweet banana peppers for this recipe.
Serves 6

- 6 hot banana peppers (AKA Hungarian or wax peppers)
- 1/2 cup Greek feta cheese, crumbled
- 2 tablespoons extra-virgin olive oil
- 2 tablespoons wine vinegar
- 1 teaspoon dried oregano

Directions

- Grill peppers until they are soft and their skins are charred, approximately 8–10 minutes; peel.
- Spread peppers flat on a serving dish; add feta over top of peppers.
- Drizzle a little olive oil and some wine vinegar over everything.
- Finish with a sprinkle of oregano, and serve.

DANDELION GREENS

Serves 6

- 4 pounds dandelion greens
- 1/2 cup extra-virgin olive oil
- 1/2 cup fresh lemon juice Salt and pepper to taste

Directions

- Cut away and discard stalks of dandelion greens; wash thoroughly.
- Bring a large pot of water to a rolling boil; add greens and stir. Cook over high heat until the greens are tender, about 8–10 minutes; remove and drain well.
- Combine olive oil, lemon juice, salt, and pepper; use as a dressing for the greens. Can be served warm or cold, as a side for grilled fish, or on their own with some crusty bread, kalamata olives, and feta. Garnish with fresh minced garlic.

SLICED TOMATO SALAD WITH FETA AND BALSAMIC VINAIGRETTE

Serves 4–6

- 4 large tomatoes, washed and sliced into round slices
- 1/4 pound Greek feta cheese, crumbled
- 1 teaspoon dried oregano
- 1/4 cup extra-virgin olive oil
- 2 tablespoons balsamic vinegar Fresh-ground black pepper

Directions

- Wash and slice tomatoes into rounds approximately 1/4-inch thick. Arrange slices in a slightly overlapping circle pattern on a large presentation platter.
- Cover tomatoes with a layer of feta cheese, making sure to spread the cheese over all the tomato slices; then sprinkle oregano over top of the cheese.
- Combine olive oil and balsamic vinegar; pour over cheese and tomatoes. Sprinkle with fresh-ground pepper and serve.

MEDITERRANEAN POULTRY RECIPES

Chicken Bruschetta

Total time: 30 minutes

Prep time: 10 minutes

Cook time: 20 minutes

Yield: 4 servings

Ingredients

- 5ml olive oil, divided
- 1 boneless, skinless chicken breast
- 80g cherry tomatoes
- 5ml balsamic vinegar
- 10g fresh basil leaves
- 1 small cloves garlic, minced
- 1 small onions, chopped

Directions

- Add half of the oil to the skillet and cook chicken over medium heat.
- In the meantime, cut basil leaves into slivers and prepare the vegetables.
- Heat the remaining oil and sauté garlic and onion for about 3 minutes.
- Stir in basil and tomatoes for about 5 minutes.

- Stir in vinegar.
- Cook until heated through and serve the chicken topped with onion and tomato mixture.

Coconut Chicken

Total time: 30 minutes

Prep time: 20 minutes

Cook time: 10 minutes

Yield: 4 servings

Ingredients

- 20g coconut, shredded
- 30g almond flour
- 1 tsp. sea salt
- 1 small egg
- 100g chicken breast, boneless, skinless
- 7.5 ml coconut oil

Directions

- In a bowl, combine shredded coconut, almond flour and sea salt.
- In a separate bowl, beat the egg; dip the chicken in the egg and roll in the flour mixture until well coated.
- Add coconut oil to a pan set over medium heat and fry the chicken until the crust begins to brown.
- Transfer the chicken to the oven and bake at 350°F for about 10 minutes.

Turkey Burgers

Total time: 25 minutes

Prep time: 15 minutes

Cook time: 10 minutes

Yield: 4 servings

Ingredients

- 1 large egg white
- 1 cup red onion, chopped
- ¾ cup fresh mint, chopped
- ½ cup dried bread crumbs
- 1 tsp. dill, dried
- ⅓ cup feta cheese, crumbled
- ¾ kg turkey, ground
- Cooking spray
- 4 hamburger buns, split
- 1 red bell pepper, roasted and cut in strips
- 2 tbsp. fresh lime juice

Directions

- Lightly beat the egg white in a bowl and add onion, mint, breadcrumbs, dill, cheese, turkey and lime juice, mix well then divide the turkey mixture into four equal burger patties.
- Spray a large nonstick skillet with cooking spray and heat on medium-high setting.
- Carefully place the patties in the skillet and cook for 8 minutes on each side or according to preference.
- Once cooked, place the burgers on the sliced buns and top with pepper strips.

Chicken with Greek Salad

Total time: 25 minutes

Prep time: 25 minutes

Cook time: 0 minutes

Yield: 4 servings

Ingredients

- 2 tbsp. extra virgin olive oil
- ⅓ cup red-wine vinegar

- 1 tsp. garlic powder
- 1 tbsp. chopped fresh dill
- ¼ tsp. sea salt
- ¼ tsp. freshly ground pepper
- 2 ½ cups chopped cooked chicken
- 6 cups chopped romaine lettuce
- 1 cucumber, peeled, seeded and chopped
- 2 medium tomatoes, chopped
- ½ cup crumbled feta cheese
- ½ cup sliced ripe black olives
- ½ cup finely chopped red onion

Directions

- In a large bowl, whisk together extra virgin olive oil, vinegar, garlic powder, dill, sea salt and pepper.
- Add chicken, lettuce, cucumber, tomatoes, feta, and olives and toss to combine well. Enjoy!

Braised Chicken with Olives

Total time: 1 hour 50 minutes

Prep time: 20 minutes

Cook time: 1 hour 30 minutes

Yield: 4 servings

Ingredients

- 1 tbsp. extra virgin olive oil
- 4 whole skinned chicken legs, cut into drumsticks and thighs
- 1 cup low-sodium canned chicken broth
- 1 cup dry white wine
- 4 sprigs thyme
- 2 tbsp. chopped fresh ginger
- 2 garlic cloves, minced
- 3 carrots, diced
- 1 medium yellow onion, diced
- 3/4¾ cup chickpeas, drained, rinsed
- ½ cup green olives, pitted and roughly chopped
- ⅓ cup raisins
- 1 cup water

Directions

- Preheat your oven to 350°F.
- Heat extra virgin olive oil in a Dutch oven or a large ovenproof skillet over medium heat.
- Add the chicken pieces into the skillet and sauté for about 5minutes per side or until browned and crisped on both sides.
- Transfer the cooked chicken to a plate and set aside.
- Lower heat to medium low and add garlic, onion, carrots, and ginger to the same skillet; cook, stirring, for about 5 minutes or until onion is translucent and tender.
- Stir in water, chicken broth, and wine; bring the mixture to a gentle boil.
- Return the chicken to the pot and stir in thyme.
- Bring the mixture back the boil and cover.
- Transfer to the oven and braise for about 45 minutes.
- Remove the pot from the oven and stir in chickpeas, olives, and raisins.
- Return to oven and braise, uncovered, for 20 minutes more.
- Remove the skillet from oven and discard thyme.

- Serve immediately.

Braised Chicken with Mushrooms and Olives

Total time: 45 minutes

Prep time: 10 minutes

Cook time: 35 minutes

Yield: 4 servings

Ingredients

- 2 ½ pounds chicken, cut into pieces
- Sea salt
- Freshly ground pepper
- 1 tbsp. plus 1 tsp. extra virgin olive oil
- 16 cloves garlic, peeled
- 10 ounces cremini mushrooms, rinsed, trimmed, and halved
- ½ cup white wine
- ⅓ cup chicken stock
- ½ cup green olives, pitted

Directions

- Heat a large skillet over medium-high heat.
- In the meantime, season the chicken with sea salt and pepper.
- Add 1 tablespoon of extra virgin olive oil to the heated skillet and add the chicken, skin side down; cook for about 6 minutes or until browned.
- Transfer to a platter and set aside.
- Add the 1 teaspoon of remaining extra virgin olive oil to the pan and sauté garlic and mushrooms for about 6 minutes or until browned.
- Add wine and bring to a gentle boil, reduce heat and cook for about 1 minute.

- Add the chicken back to the pan and stir in chicken broth and olives.
- Bring the mixture back to a gentle boil, reduce heat and simmer, covered, for about 20 minutes or until the chicken is cooked through.

Chicken with Olives, Mustard Greens, and Lemon

Total time: 40 minutes

Prep time: 10 minutes

Cook time: 30 minutes

Yield: 6 servings

Ingredients

- 2 tbsp. extra virgin olive oil, divided
- 6 skinless chicken breast halves, cut in half crosswise
- ½ cup Kalamata olives, pitted
- 1 tbsp. freshly squeezed lemon juice
- 1 1/2 pounds mustard greens , stalks removed and coarsely chopped
- 1 cup dry white wine
- 4 garlic cloves, smashed
- 1 medium red onion, halved and thinly sliced
- Sea salt
- Ground pepper
- Lemon wedges, for serving

Directions

- Heat 1 tablespoon of extra virgin olive oil in a Dutch oven or large heavy pot over medium high heat.
- Rub the chicken with sea salt and pepper and add half of it to the pot; cook, for

- about 8 minutes or until browned on all sides.
- Transfer the cooked chicken to a plate and repeat with the remaining chicken and oil.
- Add garlic and onion to the pot and lower heat to medium; cook, stirring, for about 6 minutes or until tender.
- Add chicken (with accumulated juices) and wine and bring to a boil.
- Reduce heat and cook, covered, for about 5 minutes.
- Add the greens on top of the chicken and sprinkle with sea salt and pepper.
- Cook, covered, for about 5 minutes more or until the greens are wilted and chicken is opaque.
- Remove the pot from heat and stir in olives and lemon juice.
- Serve drizzled with accumulated pan juices and garnished with lemon wedges.

Delicious Mediterranean Chicken

Total time: 55 minutes

Prep time: 25 minutes

Cook time: 30 minutes

Yield: 6 servings

Ingredients

- 2 tsp. extra virgin olive oil
- ½ cup white wine, divided
- 6 chicken breasts, skinned and deboned
- 3 cloves garlic, pressed
- ½ cup onion, chopped
- 3 cups tomatoes, chopped
- ½ cup Kalamata olives
- ¼ cup fresh parsley, chopped
- 2 tsp. fresh thyme, chopped
- Sea salt to taste

Directions

- Heat the oil and 3 tablespoons of white wine in a skillet over medium heat.
- Add the chicken and cook for about 6 minutes on each side until golden.
- Remove the chicken and put it on a plate.
- Add garlic and onions in the skillet and sauté for about 3 minutes and add the tomatoes.
- Let them cook for five minutes then lower the heat and add the remaining white wine and simmer for 10 minutes.
- Add the thyme and simmer for a further 5 minutes.
- Return the chicken to the skillet and cook on low heat until the chicken is well done.
- Add olives and parsley and cook for 1 more minute.
- Add the salt and pepper and serve.

Warm Chicken Avocado Salad

Total time: 35 minutes

Prep time: 15 minutes

Cook time: 20 minutes

Yield: 4 servings

Ingredients

- 2 tbsp. extra virgin olive oil, divided
- 500g chicken breast fillets
- 1 large avocado, peeled, diced

- 2 garlic cloves, sliced
- 1 tsp. ground turmeric
- 3 tsp. ground cumin
- 1 small head broccoli, chopped
- 1 large carrot, diced
- 1/3 cup currants
- 1 1/2 cups chicken stock
- 1 1/2 cups couscous
- Pinch of sea salt

Directions

- In a large frying pan set over medium heat, heat 1 tablespoon extra virgin olive oil; add chicken and cook for about 6 minutes per side or until cooked through; transfer to a plate and keep warm.
- In the meantime, combine currants and couscous in a heatproof bowl; stir in boiling stock and set aside, covered, for at least 5 minutes or until liquid is absorbed.
- With a fork, separate the grains.
- Add the remaining oil to a frying pan and add carrots; cook, stirring, for about 1 minute.
- Stir in broccoli for about 1 minute; stir in garlic, turmeric, and cumin.
- Cook for about 1 minute more and remove the pan from heat.
- Slice the chicken into small slices and add to the broccoli mixture; toss to combine; season with sea salt and serve with the avocado sprinkled on top.

Chicken Stew

Total time: 35 minutes

Prep time: 20 minutes

Cook time: 15 minutes

Yield: 4 servings

Ingredients

- 1 tbsp. extra virgin olive oil
- 3 chicken breast halves (8 ounces each), boneless, skinless, cut into small pieces
- Sea salt
- Freshly ground pepper
- 1 medium onion, sliced
- 4 garlic cloves, sliced
- ½ tsp. dried oregano
- 1 ½ pounds escarole, ends trimmed, chopped
- 1 cup whole-wheat couscous, cooked
- 1 (28 ounces) can whole peeled tomatoes, pureed

Directions

- In a large heavy pot or Dutch oven, heat extra virgin olive oil over medium high heat.
- Rub chicken with sea salt and pepper.
- In batches, cook chicken in olive oil, tossing occasionally, for about 5 minutes or until browned; transfer to a plate and set aside.
- Add onion, garlic and oregano, tomatoes, sea salt and pepper to the pot and cook for about 10 minutes or until onion is lightly browned.
- Add the chicken and cook, covered for about 4 minutes or until opaque.
- Fill the pot with escarole and cook for about 4 minutes or until tender.
- Serve the chicken stew over couscous.

Chicken with Roasted Vegetables

Total time: 55 minutes

Prep time: 15 minutes

Cook time: 40 minutes

Yield: 2 servings

Ingredients

- 1 large zucchini, diagonally sliced
- 250g baby new potatoes, sliced
- 6 firm plum tomatoes, halved
- 1 red onion, cut into wedges
- 1 yellow pepper, seeded and cut into chunks
- 12 black olives, pitted
- 2 chicken breast fillets, skinless, boneless
- 1 rounded tbsp. green pesto
- 3 tbsp. extra virgin olive oil

Directions

- Preheat your oven to 400ºF.
- Spread zucchini, potatoes, tomatoes, onion, and pepper in a roasting pan and scatter with olives.
- Season with sea salt and black pepper.
- Cut each chicken breast into four pieces and arrange them on top of the vegetables.
- In a small bowl, combine pesto and extra virgin olive oil and spread over the chicken. Cover with foil and cook in preheated oven for about 30 minutes.
- Uncover the pan and return to oven; cook for about 10 minutes more or until chicken is cooked through.
- Enjoy!

Grilled Chicken with Olive Relish

Total time: 21 minutes

Prep time: 15 minutes

Cook time: 6 minutes

Yield: 4 servings

Ingredients

- 4 chicken breast halves, boneless, skinless
- ¾ cup extra virgin olive oil, divided
- Sea salt
- Freshly ground black pepper
- 2 tbsp. capers, rinsed, chopped
- 1 ½ cups green olives, rinsed, pitted, and chopped
- ¼ cup lightly toasted almonds, chopped
- 1 small clove garlic, mashed with sea salt
- 1 ½ tsp. chopped fresh thyme
- 2 ½ tsp. grated lemon zest
- 2 tbsp. chopped fresh parsley

Directions

- Heat grill to high heat.
- Place 1 chicken breast on one side of a plastic wrap and drizzle with about 1 teaspoon of extra virgin olive oil and fold the wrap over the chicken.
- Pound the chicken with a heavy sauté pan or a meat mallet to about ½ inch thick.
- Repeat the process with the remaining chicken and discard the plastic wrap.
- Sprinkle chicken with sea salt and pepper and coat with about 2

tablespoons extra virgin olive oil; set aside.

- In the meantime, combine ½ cup extra virgin olive oil, capers, olives, almonds, garlic, thyme, lemon zest and parsley in a medium bowl.

- Grill the chicken for about 3 minutes per side and transfer to a cutting board.

- Let cool a bit and cut into ½-inch-thick slices.

- Arrange the chicken slices on four plates and spoon over the relish.

- Serve immediately.

Grilled Turkey with Salsa

Total time: 50 minutes

Prep time: 15 minutes

Cook time: 35 minutes

Yield: 6 servings

Ingredients

For the spice rub:

- 1 ½ tsp. garlic powder
- 1 ½ tsp. sweet paprika
- 2 tsp. crushed fennel seeds
- 2 tsp. dark brown sugar
- 1 tsp. sea salt
- 1 ½ tsp. freshly ground black pepper

For the salsa:

- 2 tbsp. drained capers
- ¼ cup pimento-stuffed green olives, chopped
- 2 scant cups cherry tomatoes, diced
- 1 ½ tbsp. extra virgin olive oil
- 1 large clove garlic, minced
- 2 tbsp. torn fresh basil leaves

- 2 tsp. fresh lemon juice
- ½ tsp. finely grated lemon zest
- 6 turkey breast cutlets
- 1 cup diced red onion
- Sea salt
- Freshly ground black pepper

Directions

- Mix together garlic powder, paprika, fennel seeds, brown sugar, salt and pepper in a small bowl.

- In another bowl, combine capers, olives, tomatoes, onion extra virgin olive oil, garlic, basil, lemon juice and zest, ¼ teaspoon sea salt and pepper; set aside.

- Grill the meat on medium high heat after dipping in the spice rub for about 3 minutes per side or until browned on both sides.

- Transfer the grilled turkey to a serving plate and let rest for about 5 minutes.

- Serve with salsa.

Curried Chicken with Olives, Apricots and Cauliflower

Total time: 8 hours 50 minutes

Refrigerator time: 8 hours

Prep time: 15 minutes

Cook time: 35 minutes

Yield: 4 to 6 servings

Ingredients

- 8 chicken thighs, skinless, boneless
- ¼ cup extra virgin olive oil, divided
- ½ tsp. ground cinnamon
- ¼ tsp. cayenne pepper
- 1 tsp. smoked paprika, divided

- 4 tsp. curry powder, divided
- 1 tbsp. apple cider vinegar
- Sea salt, to taste
- 1 head cauliflower, chopped
- 1 cup pitted green olives, halved
- ¾ cup dried apricots, chopped, soaked in hot water and drained
- ⅓ cup chopped fresh cilantro
- 6 lemon wedges

Directions

- Combine chicken thighs, 2 tablespoons extra virgin olive oil, cinnamon, cayenne, ½ teaspoon paprika, 2 tablespoons curry powder, vinegar, and sea salt in a medium bowl; toss to coat and refrigerate covered, for about 8 hours.
- Position rack in the center of oven and preheat oven to 450ºF.
- Prepare a rimmed sheet pan by lining it with parchment paper; add cauliflower and remaining olive oil, paprika, and curry powder; mix well.
- Add olives and apricots and spread the mixture in a single layer.
- Place the marinated chicken on top of the cauliflower mixture, spacing evenly apart, and roast in the preheated oven for about 35 minutes or until chicken is cooked through and cauliflower browns.
- Serve the cauliflower and chicken sprinkled with cilantro and garnished with lemon wedges.

Chicken Salad with Pine Nuts, Raisins and Fennel

Total time: 10 minutes

Prep time: 10 minutes

Cook time: 0 minutes

Chill time: 1 hour

Yield: 1 large bowl

Ingredients

For the dressing:

- 1 tbsp. extra virgin olive oil
- 3 tbsp. mayonnaise
- ½ small clove garlic, mashed with sea salt
- Pinch cayenne
- 1 tbsp. freshly squeezed fresh lemon juice

For the salad:

- 3 tbsp. chopped sweet onion
- ⅓ cup small-diced fresh fennel
- 1 cup shredded cooked chicken
- 2 tbsp. golden raisins
- 2 tbsp. toasted pine nuts
- 2 tbsp. chopped fresh flat-leaf parsley
- Sea salt
- Freshly ground pepper

Directions

- Combine extra virgin olive oil, mayonnaise, garlic, cayenne, and lemon juice in a small bowl; mix well.
- In a separate bowl, mix onion, fennel, chicken, raisins, pine nuts, and parsley; gently add in the dressing and fold the ingredients together. Season with sea salt and pepper and refrigerate for at

least 1 hour for flavors to meld before serving.

Slow Cooker Rosemary Chicken

Total time: 7 hours 20 minutes

Prep time: 20 minutes

Cook time: 7 hours, 10 minutes

Yield: 8 servings

Ingredients

- 1 small onion, thinly sliced
- 4 cloves garlic, pressed
- 1 medium red bell pepper, sliced
- 2 tsp. dried rosemary
- ½ tsp. dried oregano
- 2 pork sausages
- 8 chicken breasts, skinned, deboned and halved
- ¼ tsp. coarsely ground pepper
- ¼ cup dry vermouth
- 1 ½ tbsp. corn starch
- 2 tbsp. cold water

Directions

- Combine onion, garlic, bell pepper, rosemary and oregano in a slow cooker.
- Crumble the sausages over the mixture, casings removed.
- Arrange the chicken in a single layer over the sausage and sprinkle with pepper.
- Add the vermouth and slow-cook for 7 hours.
- Warm a deep platter, move the chicken to the platter and cover.

- Mix the cornstarch with the water in a small bowl and add this to the liquid in the slow cooker.
- Increase the heat and cover.
- Cook for about 10 minutes.

CHICKEN SOUVLAKI

Serves 6

- 2 pounds boneless, skinless chicken thighs, cut into 1-inch cubes 1/3 cup extra-virgin olive oil 2 medium onions, peeled and grated
- 4 cloves garlic, peeled and minced
- 2 tablespoons grated lemon zest
- 1 teaspoon dried oregano
- 1 teaspoon chopped fresh rosemary leaves
- 2 teaspoons salt
- 1 teaspoon pepper
- 2 tablespoons fresh lemon juice

Directions

- In a large bowl, combine the chicken, oil, onions, garlic, lemon zest, oregano, rosemary, salt, and pepper. Toss to make sure the chicken is well coated. Cover the bowl with plastic wrap and refrigerate for 8 hours or overnight. Take the chicken out of the refrigerator for 30 minutes before skewering.
- Preheat the gas or charcoal grill to medium-high. Put the chicken onto wooden or metal skewers; each skewer should hold 4 pieces.

- Place the skewers on the grill and grill for 3–4 minutes per side or until chicken is no longer pink inside.
- Drizzle lemon juice over the skewers and serve.

GREEK-STYLE ROASTED CHICKEN WITH POTATOES

Serves 4

- 4–6 Yukon gold potatoes, peeled and cut into wedges
- 1/2 cup plus 2 tablespoons extra-virgin olive oil, divided 2 tablespoons Dijon mustard
- 21/2 teaspoons salt, divided 1 teaspoon pepper, divided
- 1 teaspoon dried oregano
- 3 tablespoons fresh lemon juice, divided
- 1/2 cup hot water
- 1 (3-pound) whole chicken, rinsed and dried
- 3 cloves garlic, peeled and smashed
- 3 sprigs fresh thyme plus
- 1/2 teaspoon dried thyme 3 sprigs fresh parsley
- 1/2 large lemon, quartered
- 1/2 teaspoon dried oregano

Directions

- Preheat the oven to 375°F. Put the potatoes, 1/2 cup of oil, mustard, 1 teaspoon of salt, 1/2 teaspoon of pepper, oregano, 2 tablespoons of lemon juice, and hot water in a roasting pan. Toss the ingredients together to coat the potatoes. Reserve.

- Into the chicken cavity, put the garlic, thyme sprigs, parsley, and lemon. Combine the remaining oil and lemon juice, and rub the mixture all over the surface of the chicken. Season the chicken with the remaining salt and pepper and then sprinkle with the dried thyme and oregano.
- Place the chicken on the potatoes in the roasting pan. Roast on the middle rack for 90 minutes or until the internal temperature of the chicken reaches 180°F. Let the chicken rest for 15 minutes before serving.
- Serve warm with the roasted potatoes.

ROAST CHICKEN WITH OKRA

Serves 4

- 1 (3-pound) whole chicken, cut into pieces, rinsed and dried
- 2 teaspoons salt, divided
- 3/4 teaspoon pepper, divided
- 1/2 cup extra-virgin olive oil
- 2 large onions, peeled and sliced
- 1 pound fresh okra, rinsed and stems trimmed
- 4 large ripe tomatoes, skinned and grated
- 5 or 6 cloves garlic, peeled and sliced
- 4 or 5 whole allspice berries
- 1/2 cup chopped fresh parsley

Directions

- Season chicken with 1 teaspoon of salt and 1/2 teaspoon of pepper.

- Put the chicken in a large pot over medium-high heat with enough water to just cover it. Bring the water to a boil, reduce the heat to medium-low, and cook for 30 minutes. Skim the fat off the surface of the water and discard the fat. Remove the chicken from the pot and reserve the liquid. Preheat the oven to 375°F.

- Heat the oil in a large skillet over medium heat for 30 seconds. Add the onions and cook for 7–10 minutes or until they are translucent. Add the okra and cook for 5 minutes. Add the tomatoes, garlic, allspice, and parsley, and cook for 5 minutes. Add just enough of the reserved liquid to cover the okra.

- Transfer the contents of the skillet to a large baking dish. Place the chicken pieces on top and season with the remaining salt and pepper. Cover the baking dish.

- Bake for 30 minutes. Uncover and bake for another 15 minutes. Allow the chicken to rest for 5–10 minutes before serving.

CHICKEN CACCIATORE

Serves 4

- 1 (3-pound) whole chicken, cut into 8 pieces, rinsed and dried
- 2 teaspoons salt, divided
- 1 teaspoon pepper, divided
- 1/4 cup all-purpose flour
- 1/4 cup extra-virgin olive oil
- 1 (6-inch) Italian sausage, casing removed and crumbled
- 2 medium onions, chopped
- 1 large carrot, peeled and chopped
- 1 stalk celery, trimmed and chopped
- 1/3 cup diced green pepper, stemmed and seeded
- 1 cup sliced cremini mushrooms
- 3 bay leaves
- 2 teaspoons chopped fresh rosemary
- 1/4 cup chopped fresh parsley
- 1 tablespoon tomato paste
- 4 cloves garlic, peeled and smashed
- 1 cup dry white wine
- 1 (28-ounce) can whole tomatoes, hand crushed
- 1/2 cup hot Chicken or Turkey Stock

Directions

- Season the chicken with 1 teaspoon of salt and 1/2 teaspoon of pepper. Dredge the chicken in the flour. Set aside.

- Heat the oil in a Dutch oven (or heavy-bottomed pot) over medium-high heat for 30 seconds. Add the chicken and brown for 3–4 minutes on each side. Remove the chicken and reserve.

- Add the sausage to the pot and brown for 2 minutes. Lower the heat to medium and add the onions, carrots, celery, peppers, mushrooms, bay leaves, and rosemary. Cook the ingredients for 5–7 minutes or until the onions are translucent. Add the parsley, tomato paste, and garlic, and cook for 2 minutes. Add the wine and cook for 5–7 minutes. Add the tomatoes and stock, and cook for 2 minutes.

- Put the chicken back in the pot and lower the heat to medium-low. Partially cover the pot and cook for 60–80 minutes or until the sauce is thick and chunky. Remove the bay leaves.
- Allow the chicken to rest for 5–10 minutes before serving with the sauce.

CHICKEN GIOULBASI

Serves 4

- 1 (3-pound) whole chicken, rinsed and dried
- 1⁄4 cup extra-virgin olive oil
- 1 tablespoon grated lemon zest
- 3 tablespoons fresh lemon juice
- 11⁄2 teaspoons salt
- 1⁄2 teaspoon pepper
- 1⁄2 teaspoon sweet paprika
- 2 teaspoons dried oregano
- 6 or 7 cloves garlic, peeled and smashed
- 3⁄4 cup cubed kefalotyri or Romano cheese
- 1⁄2 large lemon, cut into wedges

Directions

- Preheat the oven to 400°F. Take two pieces of parchment paper (each 2 feet long) and lay them on a work surface in a cross pattern. Place the chicken in the middle of the parchment paper.
- In a small bowl, combine the oil, lemon zest, and lemon juice. Rub the oil-lemon mixture all over the chicken. Season the chicken with salt and pepper, and sprinkle with paprika and oregano. Place

the garlic, cheese, and lemon wedges in the cavity of the chicken.

- Wrap the parchment around the chicken, so it is completely enclosed. Use butcher's twine and tie the chicken into a bundle.
- Place the chicken in a roasting pan and roast for 90–110 minutes or until the internal temperature of the chicken is 180°F.
- Let the chicken rest for 15 minutes before unwrapping it; then serve.

GRAPE-LEAF CHICKEN STUFFED WITH FETA

Serves 4

- 1⁄2 cup crumbled feta cheese 2 scallions, ends trimmed and finely chopped
- 4 sun-dried tomatoes, finely chopped
- 1 tablespoon chopped fresh lemon verbena or lemon thyme
- 3⁄4 teaspoon pepper
- 4 boneless, skinless chicken breasts
- 11⁄2 teaspoons salt
- 8 large jarred grape leaves, rinsed and stems removed
- 1⁄4 cup extra-virgin olive oil

Directions

- Preheat the oven to 375°F. In a medium bowl, combine the feta, scallions, tomatoes, lemon verbena, and pepper. Mash the ingredients with a fork and set them aside.
- Using a sharp knife, cut a slit 3 inches wide in the middle of the thickest part of

the chicken breast. The slit should penetrate two-thirds of the way into the chicken breast to create a pocket. Stuff one-quarter of the filling into the pocket. Repeat with the remaining chicken breasts. Season the chicken with salt.

- Place 2 or 3 grape leaves on a work surface and place the chicken breast on top. Wrap the leaves around the chicken. Set the chicken, seam-side down, on a baking sheet lined with parchment paper. Brush the wrapped chicken on both sides with the oil. Repeat with the remaining chicken.

- Bake on the middle rack for 20–25 minutes. Let the chicken rest for 5 minutes before slicing each breast and serving.

GRILLED WHOLE CHICKEN UNDER A BRICK

Serves 4

- 8 cloves garlic, peeled and minced
- 1 small onion, peeled and grated
- 2 1/4 teaspoons salt, divided
- 2 tablespoons fresh lemon juice
- 2 bay leaves, crushed
- 2 teaspoons sweet paprika
- 1/4 cup Metaxa brandy or any other brandy
- 2 teaspoons chopped fresh rosemary leaves
- 2 tablespoons extra-virgin olive oil
- 1 (4-pound) whole chicken, rinsed, dried, and spatchcocked

Directions

- In a medium bowl, whisk the garlic, onion, 1/4 teaspoon of salt, lemon juice, bay leaves, paprika, brandy, rosemary, and oil.

- Pierce the chicken several times with a sharp knife to help the marinade penetrate the chicken. Place the chicken in a glass baking dish just big enough to contain it. Pour the marinade over the chicken and rub it in. Cover the baking dish with plastic wrap and refrigerate the chicken for 3–4 hours. Take the chicken out of the marinade and season it with the remaining salt.

- Preheat a gas or charcoal grill (with a lid) to medium-high. Wrap 2 heavy bricks individually in aluminum foil. Place the chicken breast-side down on the grill. Place the bricks on the chicken to weigh down the chicken as it grills. Grill the chicken for 10 minutes. Carefully remove the bricks with thick oven mitts. Flip the chicken over and place it on a side of the grill that has indirect heat. Close the grill lid and roast the chicken for 30–40 minutes or until the internal temperature reaches 180°F.

- Let the chicken rest 10 minutes before serving.

SKILLET CHICKEN PARMESAN

Serves 4

- 2/3 cup cornmeal
- 1/3 cup all-purpose flour
- 1 teaspoon dried oregano

- 1 teaspoon finely chopped and 1 cup chopped fresh basil, divided 1 teaspoon finely chopped fresh rosemary
- 4 boneless, skinless chicken breasts or thighs
- 1/2 cup plus 3 tablespoons extra-virgin olive oil, divided 1 teaspoon salt, divided
- 1/2 teaspoon pepper, divided 1 medium onion, peeled and diced
- 5 or 6 cloves garlic, peeled and minced
- 3 cups canned whole tomatoes, hand crushed
- 1/4 cup dry white wine 2 cups grated mozzarella cheese

Directions

- In a large bowl, combine the cornmeal, flour, oregano, 1 teaspoon of finely chopped basil, and rosemary. Reserve.
- Using a heavy pot or kitchen mallet, pound the chicken to 1/2-inch thickness. Cut the chicken pieces in half. Brush the pieces with 3 tablespoons of oil and season with 1/2 teaspoon of salt and 1/4 teaspoon of pepper. Dredge the chicken in the reserved cornmeal and flour mixture.
- Heat 1/4 cup oil in a large skillet over medium-high heat for 30 seconds. Add the chicken (in batches) and fry for 2–3 minutes a side or until browned. Place the chicken on a tray lined with paper towels to soak up excess oil. Discard the oil used for frying and wipe the skillet clean.

- Heat the remaining oil in the skillet over medium heat for 30 seconds. Add the onions and garlic and cook for 5–6 minutes. Add the tomatoes and wine. Increase the heat to medium-high and bring the sauce to a boil; then reduce the heat to medium-low. Season with the remaining salt and pepper. Nestle the chicken into the sauce. Cover the skillet, and cook for 30 minutes or until the sauce has thickened and chicken is tender.
- Stir in the remaining basil and top the sauce with cheese. Cover the skillet and let the cheese melt for 2 minutes. Serve warm.

CHIANTI CHICKEN

Serves 4

- 3 cloves garlic, peeled and minced
- 2 tablespoons finely chopped lemon verbena or lemon thyme 2 tablespoons finely chopped fresh parsley
- 2 1/4 teaspoons salt, divided 1/3 cup and 2 tablespoons extra-virgin olive oil, divided 4 chicken quarters (legs and thighs), rinsed and dried 3/4 teaspoon pepper 4 tablespoons unsalted butter, divided
- 2 cups red grapes (in clusters)
- 1 medium red onion, peeled and sliced
- 1 cup Chianti red wine
- 1 cup Chicken or Turkey Stock or Basic Vegetable Stock (see recipes in Chapter 2)

Directions

- Preheat the oven to 400°F. In a small bowl, whisk the garlic, lemon verbena, parsley, 1⁄4 teaspoon of salt, and 2 tablespoons of oil.

- Season the chicken with the remaining salt and pepper. Place your finger between the skin and meat of the chicken thigh and loosen it by moving your finger back and forth to create a pocket. Spread one quarter of the garlic-herb mixture into the pocket. Repeat the process with the remaining chicken quarters.

- Heat the remaining oil and 2 tablespoons of butter in a large oven-safe pot over medium-high heat for 30 seconds. Add the chicken quarters and brown them for 3–4 minutes per side.

- Top the chicken with the grapes. Roast the chicken on the middle rack of the oven for 20–30 minutes or until the chicken's internal temperature reaches 180°F. Remove the chicken and grapes from the pot and keep them warm. Remove any excess fat from the pot.

- Return the pot to the stovetop over medium heat; add the onions and cook for 3–4 minutes. Add the wine and stock, and increase the heat to medium-high. Bring the mixture to a boil, and then reduce the heat to medium-low. Cook the sauce until it thickens. Take the pot off the heat and stir in the remaining butter.

- To serve, put some of the sauce on the bottom of a plate and top with the chicken and grapes. Serve this dish with extra sauce on the side.

CHICKEN BREASTS WITH SPINACH AND FETA

Serves 4

- 1⁄2 cup frozen spinach, thawed, excess water squeezed out 4 tablespoons chopped fresh chives
- 4 tablespoons chopped fresh dill
- 1⁄2 cup crumbled feta cheese
- 1⁄3 cup ricotta cheese
- 4 boneless, skinless chicken breasts
- 1 1⁄2 teaspoons salt
- 1⁄2 teaspoon pepper
- 1⁄2 teaspoon sweet paprika
- 2 tablespoons extra-virgin olive oil
- 2 tablespoons unsalted butter
- 1⁄2 cup dry white wine
- 2 tablespoons minced red onions
- 1 clove garlic, peeled and smashed
- 2 tablespoons all-purpose flour
- 1 cup Chicken or Turkey Stock
- 1⁄3 cup heavy cream

Directions

- In a medium bowl, combine the spinach, chives, dill, feta, and ricotta. Reserve.

- Using a sharp knife, cut a 3-inch slit into the middle of the thickest part of the chicken breast. The slit should penetrate two-thirds of the way into the chicken breast to create a pocket. Stuff one-quarter of the spinach-cheese filling into the pocket. Secure the opening with toothpicks. Repeat with the remaining chicken. Then season the chicken with salt, pepper, and paprika.

- Heat the oil and butter in a large skillet over medium-high heat for 30 seconds. Brown the chicken for 3–4 minutes per side. Set the chicken aside and keep it warm. Add the wine to the skillet, and deglaze the pan. Cook for 2 minutes, or until most of the wine has evaporated. Reduce the heat to medium, and stir in the onions, garlic, and flour. Cook for 2 minutes.

- Add the stock, increase the heat to medium-high, and bring the sauce to a boil. Reduce the heat to medium and return the chicken to the skillet. Cover the skillet and cook for 25 minutes. Remove the chicken again and keep it warm. Add the cream and cook until the sauce thickens. Adjust the seasoning with more salt and pepper, if necessary.

- Slice the chicken and put it on the plates. Pour the sauce over the chicken and serve the extra sauce on the side.

CHICKEN TAGINE WITH PRESERVED LEMONS AND OLIVES

Serves 4

- 3 cloves garlic, chopped
- 1 tablespoon chopped fresh ginger
- 1½ preserved lemons, divided 4 medium onions (2 peeled and chopped, 2 peeled and sliced), divided 1 small chili pepper
- 1 tablespoon sweet paprika
- ½ teaspoon ground cumin 2 teaspoons salt, divided
- 2 tablespoons plus 1 cup chopped fresh cilantro
- 2 tablespoons chopped fresh parsley
- ¼ teaspoon saffron threads, soaked in ½ cup hot water
- ½ cup extra-virgin olive oil
- 3 bay leaves
- 4 chicken quarters (legs and thighs), rinsed and dried 2 ripe tomatoes (1 chopped and 1 sliced), divided 2 large potatoes, peeled and cut into wedges
- 1 cup water
- ½ cup pitted green olives

Directions

- To a food processor, add the garlic, ginger, ½ preserved lemon, chopped onions, chili, paprika, cumin, 1 teaspoon salt, 2 tablespoons cilantro, parsley, saffron soaked in water, oil, and bay leaves. Process until everything is chopped and well incorporated. Set the marinade aside.

- In a large bowl, combine the chicken and half of the marinade. Toss the chicken to coat it well in the marinade. Season the chicken with the remaining salt.

- In the tagine base (or Dutch oven), put the chopped tomatoes, potatoes, sliced onions, and remaining marinade. Toss to combine and coat the vegetables in the marinade. Add the water to the vegetables and stir. Place the chicken on top of the vegetables. Top the chicken with the tomato slices. Sprinkle with the olives and 1 cup cilantro. Cut the remaining lemon into six wedges and arrange them in the tagine.

- Cover the tagine and place it on the stove over medium-low heat. Cook for 45–50 minutes. Do not stir or uncover the tagine while it is cooking.
- Remove the bay leaves; serve the dish in the tagine at the table.

POMEGRANATE-GLAZED CHICKEN

Serves 4

- 4 bone-in skinless chicken breasts, rinsed and dried 1 teaspoon salt
- 1⁄2 teaspoon pepper
- 2 cups pomegranate juice
- 1⁄8 teaspoon ground mastiha
- 2 teaspoons grated orange zest
- 3 cloves garlic, peeled and smashed
- 1 teaspoon dried rosemary

Directions

- Preheat the oven to 375°F. Season the chicken with the salt and pepper. Place the chicken on a baking sheet lined with parchment paper. Bake the chicken on the middle rack in the oven for 25–30 minutes or until the chicken's internal temperature is 180°F.
- In a small pan over medium-high heat, combine the pomegranate juice, mastiha,

orange zest, garlic, and rosemary. Bring the mixture to a boil, reduce the heat to medium-low, and cook until the sauce reduces to 1⁄4 cup and has a syrup-like consistency. Remove the garlic and take the sauce off the heat.

- Brush the chicken with the reserved sauce and serve the remaining sauce on the side.

CHICKEN MASKOULI

Serves 4

- 4 chicken quarters (legs and thighs), rinsed and dried 2 teaspoons salt, divided
- 1 teaspoon pepper, divided
- 1⁄2 cup extra-virgin olive oil, divided 2 large onions, peeled and sliced
- 4 or 5 cloves garlic, minced
- 2 cups sliced cremini mushrooms
- 3 bay leaves
- 2 teaspoons thyme leaves
- 1 cup Riesling wine or other sweet white wine
- 2 cups Basic Vegetable Stock or Chicken or Turkey Stock
- 1 teaspoon sweet paprika
- 3⁄4 cup chopped walnuts or almonds
- 1⁄4 cup chopped fresh parsley

Directions

- Season the chicken with 1 teaspoon of salt and 1⁄2 teaspoon of pepper. Heat 1⁄4 cup of oil in a large skillet over medium-high heat for 30 seconds. Add the chicken quarters, and brown them for 3–

4 minutes per side. Remove the chicken and keep warm.

- Reduce the heat to medium and add the onions, garlic, mushrooms, bay leaves, and thyme. Cook for 5 minutes, and season the vegetables with the remaining salt and pepper. Cover the skillet and cook for 5 minutes.

- Remove the cover and cook for another 5 minutes or until almost all of the water has evaporated.

- Add the wine, stock, and paprika. Increase the heat to medium-high and bring the sauce to a boil. Reduce the heat to medium-low. Add the chicken back to the skillet. Cook for 35–40 minutes. The sauce will reduce and thicken.

- Put the walnuts and remaining oil in a food processor. Process until the walnuts are ground. When the chicken has finished cooking, remove it and place it on a serving platter. Add the walnut mixture to the sauce, and cook for another 5 minutes. Adjust the seasoning with more salt and pepper, if necessary. Stir in the parsley. Remove the bay leaves.

- Spoon the sauce over the chicken and serve the remaining sauce on the side.

PESTO-BAKED CHICKEN WITH CHEESE

Serves 6

- 6 skinless chicken quarters (legs and thighs), rinsed and dried

- 1/4 cup all-purpose flour
- 1/2 cup Basil and Pine Nut Pesto
- 1 teaspoon salt
- 1/2 teaspoon pepper
- 1 cup grated mozzarella cheese

Directions

- Preheat the oven to 375°F. Dredge the chicken in flour. In a large bowl, combine the chicken and Basil and Pine Nut Pesto, and toss the chicken to coat it completely.

- Place the chicken on a baking sheet lined with parchment paper. Season chicken with salt and pepper, and cover loosely with foil. Bake for 45–55 minutes or until the chicken's internal temperature is 180°F.

- Remove the foil and top the chicken with the cheese. Turn the oven to broil and broil the chicken until the cheese is melted. Serve warm.

ROSEMARY CHICKEN THIGHS AND LEGS WITH POTATOES

Serves 6

- 2 pounds chicken thighs and legs, rinsed and dried 1 leek, ends trimmed, thoroughly cleaned, cut lengthwise, and sliced 8 cloves garlic, peeled and minced
- 2 tablespoons chopped fresh rosemary
- 6 small red potatoes, halved
- 1 tablespoon extra-virgin olive oil
- 2 teaspoons salt
- 3/4 teaspoon pepper
- 1/4 cup capers

Directions

- Preheat the oven to 375°F.
- In a large baking dish, combine all the ingredients except for the capers. Toss well to combine the marinade and coat the chicken and potatoes.
- Bake in the middle rack of the oven for 1 hour or until the chicken's internal temperature is 180°F.
- Sprinkle with capers and serve.

ROAST TURKEY

Serves 10

- 1 (12-pound) turkey, cavity and neck empty, rinsed and dried 3 bay leaves
- 12 peppercorns
- 3 cloves garlic, peeled and smashed
- 6 sprigs fresh thyme plus
- 1⁄2 teaspoon thyme leaves
- 1⁄2 cup chopped fresh parsley
- 1⁄2 cup Moscato wine or other fortified wine
- 10 allspice berries
- 1⁄2 cup orange juice 1 cup plus
- 2 teaspoons salt, divided
- 1⁄4 cup extra-virgin olive oil
- 1 teaspoon pepper
- 1⁄2 teaspoon sweet paprika
- 1 teaspoon garlic powder
- 1 teaspoon chopped fresh rosemary

Directions

- In a pot or pail just large enough to hold the turkey, add the turkey and just enough cold water to cover the turkey. Take the turkey out and set it aside.

- To the water, add the bay leaves, peppercorns, garlic, thyme sprigs, parsley, wine, allspice, orange juice, and 1 cup of salt. Stir the brine until all the salt dissolves, which could take a few minutes. Place the turkey in the brine and cover it. Put the turkey and the brine in the refrigerator for 24 hours.
- Preheat the oven to 325°F. Remove the turkey from the brine, discard the brine, and let the turkey come to room temperature for 1 hour. Rinse the turkey and pat it dry with paper towels. Place the turkey on the rack of a large roaster. Rub the oil all over the turkey and then season it evenly with the remaining salt, pepper, paprika, and garlic powder. Sprinkle the turkey with the thyme leaves and rosemary.
- Roast the turkey on the middle rack for 31⁄2 hours. If the skin is getting too brown, cover the bird with aluminum foil. The internal temperature of the turkey should be 180°F (check using a meat thermometer inserted into its thigh without touching the bone).
- Remove the turkey from the oven and tent it with aluminum foil. Allow the turkey to rest for 45 minutes before serving.

TURKEY BREAST PICCATA

Serves 6

- 11⁄2 pounds whole boneless, skinless turkey breast
- 1⁄4 cup all-purpose flour
- 1⁄4 cup extra-virgin olive oil

- 1/4 cup dry white wine
- 3 tablespoons fresh lemon juice
- 1/2 cup turkey or Chicken or Turkey Stock
- 1/2 tablespoon capers
- 1/4 cup chopped fresh parsley

Directions

- Slice the turkey breast into thin scallopine-size portions and dredge in the flour.
- Heat the oil in a large skillet over medium-high heat for 30 seconds. Add the turkey and brown the slices for 2 minutes on each side.
- Add the wine and lemon juice, and let the liquid reduce by half. Add the stock and cook for 5–6 minutes or until the sauce thickens.
- To serve, sprinkle the sliced turkey with the capers and parsley, and then drizzle the sauce over the slices.

BACON-WRAPPED QUAIL

Serves 4

- 1/2 cup extra-virgin olive oil, divided 3 or 4 cloves garlic, peeled and minced
- 1/2 tablespoon grated lemon zest
- 2 tablespoons fresh lemon juice
- 1 tablespoon grated orange zest
- 1 teaspoon sweet paprika
- 1/2 teaspoon ground cinnamon 2 teaspoons fresh thyme leaves
- 1 teaspoon salt
- 1/2 teaspoon pepper 4 (7-ounce) whole quail, rinsed and dried

- 8 strips bacon
- 1 large lemon, cut into wedges

Directions

- In a large baking dish, combine 1/4 cup of oil, garlic, lemon zest, lemon juice, orange zest, paprika, cinnamon, thyme, salt, and pepper. Mix to combine the ingredients well. Add the quail and toss to coat them in the marinade. Cover the quail with plastic wrap and refrigerate them for 6 hours.
- Let the quail come to room temperature. To help the quail roast evenly, tuck each quail's wingtips back under the bird and tie the legs together with butcher's twine.
- Preheat the oven to 400°F. Wrap each quail with two strips of bacon, and tuck the ends of the bacon underneath the bird. Heat the remaining oil in a large cast-iron pan for 1 minute. Add the quail and brown them on all sides.
- Roast the quail in the cast-iron pan on the middle rack for 20 minutes. Let them rest for 5 minutes before serving with lemon wedges.

ROASTED CORNISH HENS STUFFED WITH GOAT CHEESE AND FIGS

Serves 4

- 4 Cornish hens, rinsed and dried
- 1 cup plus 1 teaspoon salt, divided
- 1/2 cup plus 2 tablespoons extra-virgin olive oil, divided 1/4 cup dry white wine 4 cloves garlic, peeled and minced

- 1 teaspoon ground fennel seeds
- 1 tablespoon sweet paprika
- 1½ tablespoons grated lemon zest, divided
- 3 tablespoons fresh lemon juice
- 3 tablespoons plus 1 teaspoon fresh thyme leaves, divided
- 1 teaspoon pepper
- ¾ cup goat cheese, crumbled
- 10 dried figs, roughly chopped
- 1 large egg, beaten

Directions

- In a pot or pail large enough to hold the hens, add the hens and just enough cold water to cover them. Take the hens out and set them aside. Add 1 cup of salt to the water, stirring until all the salt dissolves. This could take a few minutes. Place the hens in the brine and cover them. Put the hens and brine in the refrigerator overnight.
- In a large baking dish, combine the hens, ¼ cup of oil, wine, garlic, fennel, paprika, 1 tablespoon of lemon zest, lemon juice, 3 tablespoons
- thyme, remaining salt, and pepper. Toss to combine and coat the hens in the marinade. Refrigerate the hens for 3 hours. Let the hens come to room temperature for 30 minutes in the marinade then discard marinade. Preheat the oven to 400°F.
- In a bowl, combine the goat cheese, remaining oil, remaining thyme, figs, remaining lemon zest, and egg. Stir well

to combine the filling. Stuff each hen with one-quarter of the cheese stuffing. Tie the legs together with butcher's twine.

- Place the hens in a roasting pan (raised on a rack) and pour the excess marinade over them. Roast the hens on the middle rack for 1 hour or until their internal temperature is 180°F.
- Tent the hens with aluminum foil and let them rest for 10 minutes before serving them.

ROAST LEMON CHICKEN

Serves 4
- 1 whole chicken
- Salt and pepper to taste
- Juice of 2 lemons, shells retained
- 2 tablespoons extra-virgin olive oil
- 1 tablespoon prepared mustard
- 1 teaspoon dried oregano

Directions

- Preheat the oven to 400°F.
- Wash the chicken well inside and out and pat dry. Sprinkle inside and out with salt and pepper, and stuff the squeezed-out lemon halves into the cavity. Place chicken breast down on a rack in a shallow roasting dish. Combine lemon juice, olive oil, mustard, and oregano; brush/pour over entire chicken.
- Bake for 60–70 minutes, making sure to turn chicken over at halfway point and basting it regularly with juices from pan.
- To test if it's done, prick with a fork and see if juices run clear, or test with a meat

thermometer for 165°F. When done, turn off the oven and cover chicken in aluminum foil. Let rest in a warm oven for 10 minutes.

- Serve hot with pan juices.

CHICKEN WITH YOGURT

Serves 4

- 1 whole chicken
- 2 lemons, halved
- Salt and pepper
- 2 cups strained yogurt
- 2 tablespoons milk
- 2 tablespoons fresh mint, chopped
- 2 cups dry bread crumbs
- 1/2 cup salted butter

Directions

- Preheat the oven to 350°F.
- Wash chicken well inside and out and pat dry with a paper towel. Cut chicken into sections; rub vigorously with lemon halves and sprinkle with salt and pepper. Place pieces in a colander; let stand for 1 hour.
- Place yogurt in a mixing bowl. Add milk and mint; mix well with a whisk until smooth.
- Dip each piece of chicken into yogurt mix, then cover entirely with a good sprinkling of bread crumbs. Place on a greased roasting pan; drizzle melted butter over the top.
- Bake for about 1 hour, until the chicken pieces are golden brown.

- Serve with a side of rice or fried potatoes.

CHICKEN WITH EGG NOODLES AND WALNUTS

Serves 4–6

- 1 whole chicken
- 1/2 cup extra-virgin olive oil 1 onion, diced
- 1/4 cup butter 2 cups tomato pulp, minced and sieved
- 4 cups boiling water
- 1 tablespoon fresh mint, chopped
- Salt and pepper
- 1 pound square egg noodles (Greek hilopites)
- 1/2 cup crushed walnuts Grated myzithra or Parmesan cheese for garnish (optional)

Directions

- Wash chicken well inside and out and pat dry with a paper towel. Cut into sections.
- Heat oil. Sauté onion slightly; add butter and chicken and sauté thoroughly on all sides.
- Add tomatoes, boiling water, mint, salt, and pepper. Bring to a boil; cover and simmer over medium-low heat for 30 minutes.
- Add egg noodles and crushed walnuts; give a good stir. Cover and continue to simmer for another 30 minutes.

- Stir before serving hot with some grated myzithra or Parmesan cheese over each helping.

STUFFED GRILLED CHICKEN BREASTS

Serves 6

- 6 large boneless, skinless chicken breasts
- 1 cup crumbled Greek feta cheese
- 1/2 cup finely minced sun-dried tomatoes
- 1 teaspoon dried oregano
- 2 tablespoons extra-virgin olive oil
- Salt and pepper

Directions

- Wash chicken breasts well and pat dry with a paper towel.
- In a bowl, mix feta with sun-dried tomatoes and oregano; combine thoroughly.
- Place each chicken breast on a flat surface; using a sharp paring knife, carefully slit the top edge of each breast and make a deep incision that runs within the length of each breast. Be careful not to pierce any holes that would allow stuffing to seep out while grilling.
- Use a small spoon to stuff an equal portion of cheese mixture into each breast; use poultry pins or toothpicks to close openings.
- Sear breasts in a heated frying pan with olive oil, approximately 2–3 minutes per side.

- Sprinkle with salt and pepper; cook on a prepared grill over high heat for about 15 minutes, approximately 8 minutes per side. Serve immediately.

CHICKEN LIVERS IN RED WINE

Serves 4

- 1 pound chicken livers
- 1 cup chicken broth
- 1/2 cup butter 1 small onion, diced
- 1 tablespoon all-purpose flour
- 1/2 cup red wine Salt and pepper
- 2 tablespoons fresh parsley, finely chopped

Directions

- Wash chicken livers thoroughly and drain well before using. Bring broth to a boil in a small pan and let simmer over low heat.
- Melt butter in another frying pan. Slightly sauté onion; add chicken livers and cook over high heat for 3–5 minutes, stirring constantly to avoid browning.
- Sprinkle flour over top of livers and butter; continue to stir well to form a sauce in the bottom of the pan. Stir constantly to avoid clumping.
- Slowly add hot broth to the pan with the livers, stirring constantly. Turn heat to high and slowly add wine; continue to simmer and stir several minutes. Reduce heat to low; cook for another 5–10 minutes to thicken sauce.

- Season with salt and pepper and serve hot with chopped parsley as a garnish over a bed of mashed potatoes.

CHICKEN GALANTINE

Serves 6

- 1 small whole chicken
- 1 shallot
- 2 cloves garlic
- 1⁄4 cup pistachio nuts 8 dates
- 1⁄2 pound ground chicken 1 egg white
- 1 teaspoon dried oregano
- 1 teaspoon dried marjoram
- Fresh-cracked black pepper, to taste
- Kosher salt, to taste

Directions

- Preheat the oven to 325°F.
- Carefully remove all the skin from the chicken by making a slit down the back and loosening the skin with your fingers (keep the skin intact as much as possible); set aside the chicken and the skin. Remove the breast from bone. Chop the shallot and mince the garlic. Chop the nuts and dates.
- Mix together the ground chicken, egg white, nuts, dates, shallots, garlic, oregano, marjoram, pepper, and salt.
- Lay out the skin, then lay the breast lengthwise at the center. Spoon the ground chicken mixture on top, and fold over the rest of skin. Place in a loaf pan and bake for 1⁄2–2 hours (when the internal temperature of the loaf reaches 170° F, it's done). Let cool, then slice.

SPICY TURKEY BREAST WITH FRUIT CHUTNEY

Serves 6

- 2 jalapeño chili peppers
- 2 cloves garlic
- 1 tablespoon olive oil
- 2 teaspoons all-purpose flour
- Fresh-cracked black pepper, to taste
- Cooking spray
- 1 1⁄2 pounds whole boneless turkey breast 1 shallot
- lemon
- 2 pears
- tablespoon honey

Directions

- Preheat the oven to 350°F.
- Stem, seed, and mince the peppers. Mince the garlic. In a blender, purée the chili peppers, garlic, and oil. Mix together the flour and black pepper.
- Spray a rack with cooking spray. Dredge the turkey in the flour mixture, then dip it in the pepper mixture, and place on rack. Cover loosely with foil and roast for 1 hour. Remove foil and brown for 10 minutes.
- While the turkey cooks, prepare the chutney: Finely dice the shallots. Juice the lemon and grate the rind for zest. Dice the pears. Mix together the pears, shallot, lemon juice, zest, and honey.
- Thinly slice the turkey, and serve with chutney.

GRILLED DUCK BREAST WITH FRUIT SALSA

Serves 6

- plum
- peach
- nectarine
- red onion
- 3 sprigs mint
- Fresh-cracked black pepper, to taste
- tablespoon olive oil
- teaspoon chili powder
- 1 1/2 pounds boneless duck breast

Directions

- Preheat the grill. Dice the plum, peach, nectarine, and onion. Mince the mint. Toss together the fruit, onion, mint, and pepper.
- Mix together the oil and chili powder. Dip the duck breast in the oil, and cook to desired doneness on grill.
- Slice duck on the bias and serve with a spoonful of salsa.

QUAIL WITH PLUM SAUCE

Serves 6

- quail 12 plums
- 2 yellow onions
- 1 stalk celery
- 1 carrot
- 1/4 cup olive oil 2 bay leaves
- 1 cup dry red wine
- 1 quart Hearty Red Wine Brown Stock
- 2 sprigs thyme, leaves only
- 1/2 bunch parsley stems Kosher salt, to taste Fresh-cracked black pepper, to taste .

Directions

- Cut the quail in half and remove breast and back bones (reserve bones). Peel, pit, and chop the plums. Chop the onions and celery. Peel and chop the carrot.
- Heat the oil to medium-high temperature in a large stockpot. Brown the quail bones, then add the onions, carrots, and celery, and brown slightly. Add the plums and wine, and let reduce by half.
- Add the stock and herbs; simmer for 6 hours, then strain, removing bay leaves.
- Preheat grill.
- Season the quail meat with the salt and pepper; grill on each side until golden brown. Serve with stock.

SLOW-COOKED DUCK

You'll need a day's head start on this recipe. Slow-cooking makes any ingredient extremely tender.

Serves 6

- 3-pound duck
- 6 bay leaves
- 1 bunch parsley stems, chopped
- 2 tablespoons coarse salt
- 1 teaspoon black pepper
- 1/2 bunch sage 1/2 bunch thyme 1/2 cup olive oil

Directions

- Remove and discard all the skin and visible fat from the duck. Cut the duck into serving portions.
- Place the duck in a single layer on a baking sheet. Cover the duck with the herbs and spices. Wrap with plastic wrap. Refrigerate overnight. Rinse and dry thoroughly before baking.
- Preheat the oven to 250°F.
- Place the oil in a baking dish. Add the duck, cover, and bake for 8–12 hours. Allow the duck to cool for approximately 1 hour.
- Thoroughly drain off and discard the oil from the duck; remove bay leaves. Transfer the duck to a broiler pan; flash under the broiler to brown before serving.

GOOSE BRAISED WITH CITRUS

Serves 6
- 2 yellow onions
- carrot
- stalk celery
- grapefruit
- 2 oranges
- lemon
- lime
- tablespoon olive oil
- 3-pound goose
- 1⁄2 cup port wine
- 1⁄4 cup honey 2 cups Hearty Red Wine Brown Stock

Directions
- Preheat the oven to 350°F.

- Cut the onions into wedges. Peel and cut the carrot into quarters. Roughly chop the celery. Quarter the grapefruit, oranges, lemon, and lime (leave the peels on).
- Heat the oil to medium-high temperature in a large Dutch oven. Sear the goose on all sides. Add the vegetables and fruit; cook for 5 minutes, stirring constantly. Add the wine and reduce by half, then add the honey and stock. When the liquid begins to boil, cover and braise in the oven for 3–4 hours.
- Serve the cooking liquid (which will thicken as it cooks) as a sauce accompanying the goose.

SAGE-RICOTTA CHICKEN BREASTS

Serves 6
- 6 chicken breast halves with bone and skin on
- 6 fresh sage leaves
- 1⁄2 cup part-skim ricotta cheese 1 egg white
- 1⁄4 cup niçoise olives Fresh-cracked black pepper, to taste

Directions
- Preheat the oven to 375°F.
- Rinse the chicken in cold water. Using your finger, make an opening in the skin where the wing was joined and loosen the skin away from the breast. Slice the sage.

- Mix together the sage, cheese, and egg, and place this mixture in a pastry bag. Pipe the mixture under the skin through the opening you made. Place the chicken on a rack in a baking dish; roast for approximately 30– 45 minutes, until the internal temperature of the chicken reaches 165°F and the outside is browned.
- Remove pits and chop olives. After you remove the chicken from the rack, sprinkle with olives and pepper, and serve.

TURKEY TETRAZZINI

Serves 6

- 1 pound boneless, skinless turkey
- 1 leek (white part only)
- 3 cloves garlic
- 3 cups mushrooms
- 1/4 cup olive oil, divided
- 1/8 cup bread crumbs
- 1/4 cup all-purpose flour
- 1 cup skim milk
- 2 ounces Parmesan, grated
- 2 ounces Romano, grated
- Fresh-cracked black pepper, to taste

Directions

- Preheat the oven to 375°F.
- Cut the turkey into bite-size portions. Slice the leek and mince the garlic. Clean the mushrooms with a damp paper towel, then slice them. Mix half of the oil with the bread crumbs.

- Heat the remaining oil over medium heat in a medium-size saucepan; brown the turkey, then remove and keep warm. Add the leeks, garlic, and mushrooms to the pan that you cooked the turkey in; cook thoroughly, then add the flour.
- Whisk in the milk, stirring constantly to avoid lumping. Remove from heat and add the cheeses. Spoon the mixture into a casserole pan and top with bread crumb mixture; bake for 30 minutes. Season with pepper before serving.

Chicken and Penne

Total time: 50 minutes

Prep time: 20 minutes

Cook time: 30 minutes

Yield: 4 servings

Ingredients

- 1 package penne pasta
- 1 ½ tbsp. butter
- ½ cup red onion, chopped
- 2 cloves garlic, pressed
- ¾ kg chicken breasts, deboned and skinned, cut in halves
- 1 can artichoke hearts, soaked in water, chopped
- ½ cup feta cheese, crumbled
- 2 tbsp. lemon juice
- 1 tomato, chopped
- 3 tbsp. fresh parsley, chopped
- Sea salt
- Freshly ground black pepper
- 1 tsp. oregano, dried

Directions

- Cook the penne pasta until al dente in a large saucepan with salted boiling water.
- Melt butter in a large skillet over medium heat and add the onions and garlic.
- Cook these for 2 minutes and add the chicken.
- Stir occasionally until the chicken is golden brown for about 6 minutes.
- Drain the artichoke hearts and add them to the skillet together with the cheese, lemon juice, tomatoes, oregano, parsley and drained pasta.
- Reduce the heat to medium low and cook for 3 minutes.
- Add the salt and pepper to taste and serve warm.

MEDITERRANEAN SEAFOOD RECIPES

Salmon and Vegetable Kedgeree

Total time: 30 minutes
Prep time: 10 minutes
Cook time: 20 minutes

Ingredients

- 60ml basmati rice
- 7.5ml extra virgin olive oil
- 2g curry powder
- 100g skinless hot-smoked salmon portions, flaked
- 100g vegetable mix
- Sea salt and pepper, to taste
- 1 green onion, thinly sliced

Directions

- In a saucepan of boiling salted water, add rice, turn heat to low and cook, covered, until just tender, for about 12 minutes.
- Add extra virgin olive oil to a pan set over medium heat and cook the onion, stirring until tender, for about 3 minutes.
- Stir in curry powder and continue cooking until fragrant, for about 1 minute.
- Stir in rice until well combined and then add salmon, vegetables, salt and pepper.
- Continue cooking until heated through, for about 3 minutes.
- Serve.

Grilled Sardines with Wilted Arugula

Total time: 25 minutes
Prep time: 15 minutes
Cook time: 10 minutes
Servings: 4

Ingredients

- 2 large bunches baby arugula, trimmed
- 16 fresh sardines, innards and gills removed
- 2 tsp. extra virgin olive oil
- Sea salt
- Freshly ground black pepper
- Lemon wedges, for garnish

Directions

- Prepare your outdoor grill or a stove-top griddle.
- Rinse arugula under running water; shake off excess water and arrange them on a platter; set aside.

- Rinse sardines in water and rub to remove scales; wipe them dry and combine with extra virgin olive oil in a large bowl.
- Toss to coat.
- Place the sardines over the grill and grill for about 3 minutes per side or until golden brown and crispy.
- Season with sea salt and pepper and immediately transfer to the platter lined with arugula.
- Serve right away garnished with lemon wedges.

Curry Salmon with Napa Slaw

Total time: 1 hour
Prep time: 15 minutes
Cook time: 45 minutes
Yield: 4 servings

Ingredients

- 1 cup brown basmati rice
- A pinch of coarse salt
- A pinch of ground black pepper
- 1 pound (½ head) Napa cabbage, sliced crosswise
- 2 tbsp. extra virgin olive oil
- ¼ cup freshly squeezed lime juice
- ½ cup fresh mint leaves
- 1 pound carrots, coarsely grated
- 4 (6 ounces each) salmon filets
- 2 tsp. curry powder
- Lime wedges for serving

Directions

- Bring two cups of water to a gentle boil in a large saucepan set over medium-low heat; add rice and season with sea salt and pepper; turn heat to low and cook, covered, for about 35 minutes.
- In the meantime, combine Napa cabbage, extra virgin olive oil, lime juice, mint, carrots, salt and black pepper in a large bowl; toss until well combined.
- Set broiler rack 4 inches from heat and preheat it.
- Place salmon in a baking sheet lined with foil and rub it with curry, salt and pepper.
- Broil the fish for about 8 minutes or until just cooked through.
- Serve the cooked rice alongside green salad and grilled salmon.

Shrimp and Pasta

Total time: 20 minutes
Prep time: 15 minutes
Cook time: 5 minutes
Yield: 4 servings

Ingredients

- 2 tsp. extra virgin olive oil
- 2 garlic cloves, minced
- 1 pound shrimp, peeled, deveined
- 2 cups chopped plum tomato
- ¼ cup thinly sliced fresh basil
- 2 tbsp. capers, drained
- ⅓ cup chopped pitted Kalamata olives
- ¼ tsp. freshly ground black pepper
- 4 cups hot cooked angel hair pasta
- ¼ cup crumbled feta cheese
- Cooking spray

Directions

- In a large nonstick skillet set over medium high heat, heat extra virgin olive oil; add garlic and sauté for about 30 seconds.
- Add shrimp and sauté for 1 minute more.
- Stir in tomato and basil and lower heat to medium low; simmer for about 3 minutes or until the tomato is tender.
- Stir in capers, Kalamata olives and black pepper.
- In a large bowl, combine pasta and shrimp mixture; toss to mix and top with cheese.
- Serve immediately.

Roasted Fish

Total time: 40 minutes

Prep time: 10 minutes

Cook time: 30 minutes

Yields: 4 servings

Ingredients

- 1 tbsp. olive oil
- 1 (14-oz) can drained artichoke hearts
- 4 cloves garlic, crushed
- 1 green bell pepper, cut into small strips
- ½ cup halved pitted olives
- 1 pint cherry tomatoes
- 1 tbsp. fennel seed
- 1 ½ lb. cod, quartered
- 4 ½ tsp. grated orange peel
- 2 tbsp. drained capers
- ⅓ to ½ cup fresh orange juice
- A pinch ground pepper
- A pinch salt

Directions

- Preheat your oven to 450°F.
- Generously grease a 10×15-inch baking pan with 1 tablespoon olive oil.
- Arrange the artichoke hearts, garlic, bell pepper, olives, tomatoes and fennel seed in the prepared pan.
- Place the fish over the vegetables and top with orange peel, capers, orange juice, pepper and salt.

Baked Fish

Total time: 1 hour

Prep time: 10 minutes

Cook time: 50 minutes

Yields: 4 servings

Ingredients

- 2 tsp. extra virgin olive oil
- 1 large sliced onion
- 1 tbsp. orange zest
- ¼ cup orange juice
- ¼ cup lemon juice
- ¾ cup apple juice
- 1 minced clove garlic
- 1 (16 oz.) can whole tomatoes, drained and coarsely chopped, the juice reserved
- ½ cup reserved tomato juice
- 1 bay leaf
- ½ tsp. crushed dried basil
- ½ tsp. crushed dried thyme
- ½ tsp. crushed dried oregano
- 1 tsp. crushed fennel seeds
- A pinch of black pepper
- 1 lb. fish fillets (perch, flounder or sole)

Directions

- Add oil to a large nonstick skillet set over medium heat.
- Sauté the onion in the oil for about 5 minutes or until tender.
- Stir in all the remaining ingredients except the fish.
- Simmer uncovered for about 30 minutes.
- Arrange the fish in a baking dish and cover with the sauce.
- Bake the fish at 375°F, uncovered, for about 15 minutes or until it flakes easily when tested with a fork.

Spanish Cod

Total time: 35 minutes

Prep time: 20 minutes

Cook time: 15 minutes

Yield: 6 servings

Ingredients

- 1 tbsp. extra virgin olive oil
- 1 tbsp. butter
- ¼ cup onion, finely chopped
- 2 tbsp. garlic, chopped
- 1 cup tomato sauce
- 15 cherry tomatoes, halved
- ¼ cup deli marinated Italian vegetable salad, drained and chopped
- ½ cup green olives, chopped
- 1 dash cayenne pepper
- 1 dash black pepper
- 1 dash paprika
- 6 cod fillets

Directions

- Place a large skillet over medium heat and add the olive oil and butter.

- Add the onion and garlic and cook until garlic starts browning.
- Add the tomato sauce and tomatoes and let them simmer.
- Stir in the marinated vegetables, olives and spices.
- Cook the fillet in the sauce for 8 minutes over medium heat.
- Serve immediately.

Greek Salmon Burgers

Total time: 30 minutes

Prep time: 15 minutes

Cook time: 15 minutes

Yield: 4 servings

Ingredients

- 1 pound skinless salmon fillets, diced
- 1 large egg white
- ½ cup panko
- 1 pinch sea salt
- ¼ tsp. freshly ground black pepper
- ½ cup cucumber slices
- ¼ cup crumbled feta cheese
- 4 (2.5-oz) toasted ciabatta rolls

Directions

- In a food processor, combine together salmon, egg white, and panko; pulse until salmon is finely chopped.
- Form the salmon mixture into four 4-inch patties and season with sea salt and pepper.
- Heat the grill to medium high heat and cook the patties, turning once, for about 7 minutes per side or until just cooked through.

- Serve with favorite toppings (such as sliced cucumbers and feta) and buns.

Grilled Tuna

Total time: 1 hour 16 minutes

Prep time: 10 minutes

Chill time: 1 hour

Cook time: 6 minutes

Yield: 4 servings

Ingredients

- 4 tuna steaks, 1 inch thick
- 3 tbsp. extra virgin oil
- ½ cup hickory wood chips, soaked
- Sea salt
- Freshly ground black pepper
- Juice of 1 lime

Directions

- Place tuna and the olive oil in a zip lock plastic bag, seal and refrigerate for an hour.
- Prepare a charcoal or gas grill.
- When using a coal grill, scatter a handful of hickory wood chips when the coals are hot for added flavor.
- Lightly grease the grill grate.
- Season the tuna with salt and pepper and cook on the grill for about 6 minutes, turning only once.
- Transfer to a plate.
- Drizzle the lime juice over the fish and serve immediately.

Easy Fish Dish

Total time: 45 minutes

Prep time: 15 minutes

Cook time: 30 minutes

Yields: 4 servings

Ingredients

- 4 fillets halibut (6 ounces)
- 1 tbsp. Greek seasoning
- 1 tbsp. lemon juice
- ¼ cup olive oil
- ¼ cup capers
- 1 jar (5 ounce) pitted Kalamata olives
- 1 chopped onion
- 1 large tomato, chopped
- A pinch of freshly ground black pepper
  A pinch of salt

Directions

- Preheat your oven to 250°F.
- Arrange the halibut fillets onto an aluminum foil sheet and sprinkle with Greek seasoning.
- In a bowl, combine together lemon juice, olive oil, capers, olives, onion, tomato, salt and pepper; spoon the mixture over the fillets and fold the edges of the foil to seal.
- Place the folded foil onto a baking sheet and bake for about 40 minutes or until the fish flakes easily when touched with a fork.

Salmon Bean Stir-Fry

Total time: 20 minutes

Prep time: 10 minutes

Cook time: 10 minutes

Yield: 4 servings

Ingredients

- 1g crushed red pepper

- 2.5g cornstarch
- 5ml rice wine
- 7.5ml black bean-garlic sauce
- 7.5ml rice vinegar
- 30ml cup water
- 5ml canola oil
- 100g salmon, skinned, cubed
- 10g scallions, sliced
- 90g bean sprouts

Directions

- In a bowl, whisk together crushed red pepper, cornstarch, rice wine, bean-garlic sauce, vinegar and water until well combined.
- Add oil to skillet set over medium heat.
- Stir in fish and cook for about 2 minutes.
- Stir in the sauce mixture, scallions and sprouts.
- Cook for about 3 minutes or until the sprouts are tender and cooked down.

Mediterranean Flounder

Total time: 40 minutes

Prep time: 10 minutes

Cook time: 30 minutes

Yield: 4 servings

Ingredients

- 5 Roma tomatoes
- 2 tbsp. extra virgin olive oil
- ½ onion, chopped
- 2 garlic cloves, chopped
- 1 pinch Italian seasoning
- 1 lb. flounder/tilapia/halibut
- 4 tbsp. capers
- 24 Kalamata olives, pitted and chopped

- 1 tsp. freshly squeezed lemon juice
- ¼ cup white wine
- 6 leaves fresh basil, chopped; divided
- 3 tbsp. Parmesan cheese

Directions

- Preheat your oven to 425°F.
- Plunge the tomatoes into boiling water and immediately transfer them into a bowl of ice water; peel the skins and chop them
- Add extra virgin olive oil to a skillet set over medium heat and sauté onions until translucent.
- Stir in garlic, Italian seasoning, and tomatoes and cook until tomatoes are tender.
- Stir in wine, lemon juice, capers, olives, and half of basil.
- Lower heat and stir in Parmesan cheese; cook for about 15 minutes or until the mixture is bubbly and hot.
- Place fish in a baking dish and cover with the sauce; bake in the preheated oven for about 20 minutes or until fish is cooked through.

Fish with Olives, Tomatoes, and Capers

Total time: 21 minutes

Prep time: 5 minutes

Cook time: 16 minutes

Yield: 4 servings

Ingredients

- 4 tsp. extra virgin olive oil, divided
- 4 (5-ounce) sea bass fillets

- 1 small onion, diced
- ½ cup white wine
- 2 tbsp. capers
- 1 cup canned diced tomatoes, with juice
- ½ cup pitted black olives, chopped
- ¼ tsp. crushed red pepper
- 2 cups fresh baby spinach leaves
- Sea salt and pepper

Directions

- Heat 2 teaspoons of extra virgin olive oil in a large nonstick skillet set over medium high heat.
- Add fish and cook for about 3 minutes per side or until opaque in the center.
- Transfer the cooked fish to a plate and keep warm.
- Add the remaining oil to the skillet and sauté onion for about 2 minutes or until translucent.
- Stir in wine and cook for about 2 minutes or until liquid is reduced by half.
- Stir in capers, tomatoes, olives, and red pepper and cook for about 3 minutes more.
- Add spinach and cook, stirring for about 3 minutes or until silted.
- Stir in sea salt and pepper and spoon sauce over fish.
- Serve immediately.

Mediterranean Cod

Total time: 50 minutes

Prep time: 15 minutes

Cook time: 35 minutes

Yield: 4 servings

Ingredients

- 1 tbsp. extra virgin olive oil
- 100g frozen chopped onion
- 1 tbsp. frozen chopped garlic
- 230g can Italian tomatoes, chopped
- 1 tbsp. tomato purée
- 400g pack skinless and boneless cod fillets
- 200g frozen mixed peppers
- 1 tbsp. chopped frozen parsley
- 50g pitted black olives
- 800g package frozen white rice

Directions

- Add extra virgin olive oil to a saucepan set over medium heat; stir in onion and sauté for about 3 minutes.
- Add garlic and sauté for 2 minutes more or until fragrant.
- Stir in the tomatoes, tomato puree, and water and bring to a gentle boil.
- Reduce heat and simmer for about 20 minutes or until thickened.
- Add cod and peppers; nudge the fish in the sauce a bit and bring back to a boil; lower heat and simmer for about 8 minutes.
- Sprinkle with parsley and olives and simmer for 2 minutes more.
- In the meantime, follow package instructions to cook rice.
- Serve fish with hot rice.

BIANKO FROM CORFU

Serves 4

- 1/2 cup extra-virgin olive oil, divided 2 large onions, peeled and sliced
- 6 cloves garlic, peeled and minced
- 2 medium carrots, peeled and sliced
- 1 cup chopped celery
- 1 1/2 teaspoons salt, divided 1 teaspoon pepper, divided
- 4 large potatoes, peeled and cut into 1/2-inch slices
- 4 whitefish fillets (cod or grouper), skinned
- 3–5 tablespoons fresh lemon juice
- 1/4 cup chopped fresh parsley

Directions

- Heat 1/4 cup of oil in a heavy-bottomed pot over medium heat for 30 seconds. Add the onions, garlic, carrots, and celery. Cook the vegetables for 5–7 minutes or until the onions soften. Then season them with 1/2 teaspoon of salt and 1/4 teaspoon of pepper.
- Add the potatoes and the remaining salt and pepper. Add just enough hot water to cover the potatoes. Increase the heat to medium-high and bring the water to a boil. Reduce the heat to medium-low, cover the pot, leaving the lid slightly ajar, and cook for 12 minutes.
- Place the fillets over the potatoes and top with the remaining oil. Cover the fish and cook for another 12–15 minutes or until the whitefish is opaque and flaky.
- Uncover the pot and add the lemon juice. Don't stir it; shake the pot back and forth to allow the juice to penetrate the layers.

Adjust the seasoning with more salt and pepper, if necessary.
- Place the fish and potatoes on a large platter and top with the parsley. Serve immediately.

GRILLED SALMON WITH LEMON AND LIME

Serves 4

- 4 (6-ounce) salmon fillets, skins on
- 1/4 cup extra-virgin olive oil
- 1 tablespoon grated lemon zest
- 1 1/2 teaspoons grated lime zest
- 1 1/2 teaspoons salt
- 1/2 teaspoon pepper
- 3 tablespoons vegetable oil
- 1 large lemon, cut into wedges

Directions

- Preheat a gas or charcoal grill to medium-high. Brush the grill surface to make sure it is thoroughly clean. Rinse the fillets and pat them dry with a paper towel. Rub the fillets with the olive oil on both sides.
- Sprinkle both sides of the fillets with the lemon zest, lime zest, salt, and pepper.
- When the grill is ready, dip a clean tea towel in the vegetable oil and wipe the grill surface with the oil.
- Place the salmon on the grill, skin-side down, and grill for 6–7 minutes. Don't touch the fillets, just let them grill. Flip the salmon over and grill for another 2–3 minutes.
- Serve the salmon with lemon wedges.

SEA BASS BAKED WITH COARSE SEA SALT

Serves 2

- 1 pound whole sea bass, cleaned, gutted, and scaled
- 3 or 4 sprigs fresh thyme
- 1⁄2 cup chopped fresh parsley 1 large lemon, sliced
- 2 cups coarse sea salt
- 1⁄3 cup all-purpose flour
- 3 egg whites, beaten
- 1 tablespoon grated lemon zest
- 1⁄2 cup cold water
- 1⁄2 cup Ladolemono

Directions

- Preheat the oven to 450°F. Rinse fish and pat dry with a paper towel. Place thyme, parsley, and lemon slices in the cavity of the fish. Reserve the sea bass.

- In a medium bowl, combine the salt, flour, eggs, and zest. Gradually stir in the water until the mixture comes together and resembles a paste. You may not need all the water; the paste should not be too runny.

- On a baking sheet lined with parchment paper, place a layer of the salt mixture just large enough to set the entire fish on (about 1⁄3 of the salt mixture). Place the fish on top of the salt and encase it (leave the head and tail exposed) with the remaining salt mixture. Pack the salt around the sea bass so it adheres. Place the sheet on the middle rack and bake

for 30 minutes. Let the fish cool for 10 minutes.

- Using a hammer or the flat side of a meat tenderizer, carefully crack the salt crust to reveal the fish. With the back of a knife, remove the salty skin and carefully flip the fish onto a serving platter and remove the skin from the other side.

- Spoon a little of the Ladolemono sauce over the fish and serve the rest of the sauce on the side.

BEER-BATTER FISH

Serves 4

- 3⁄4 cup all-purpose flour 3⁄4 cup cornstarch
- 1 teaspoon baking powder 1¼ teaspoons salt, divided 1–1½ cups cold dark beer 4 (6-ounce) haddock or cod fillets, skins removed and cut into 3 or 4 pieces
- Sunflower oil for frying

Directions

- In a large bowl, combine the flour, cornstarch, baking powder, and 1⁄2 teaspoon of salt. Slowly stir in the beer to reach the consistency of a thin pancake batter (you might not need all the beer, so drink what's left). Place the batter in the refrigerator for an hour.

- Rinse the fish and pat it dry with a paper towel. Season the fish with 1⁄2 teaspoon of salt.

- Fill a deep frying pan with 3 inches of the oil. Over medium-high heat, bring the oil temperature to 365°F. Adjust the heat to keep the temperature at 365°F while frying. Fry the fish (in batches) for 3–4 minutes or until just golden. Transfer the fish to a tray lined with paper towels to soak up excess oil.
- Season the fish with the remaining salt and serve it immediately.

GRILLED SARDINES

Serves 4

- 2 pounds fresh sardines, heads removed, cleaned, gutted, and scaled
- 1/2 cup extra-virgin olive oil, divided 2 teaspoons salt
- 3/4 teaspoon pepper
- 3 tablespoons vegetable oil
- 3 tablespoons fresh lemon juice
- 1 1/2 teaspoons dried oregano

Directions

- Preheat a gas or charcoal grill to medium-high. Brush the grill surface to make sure it is thoroughly clean. Rinse the sardines and pat them dry with a paper towel.
- Rub the sardines on both sides with 1/4 cup of olive oil. Sprinkle both sides with salt and pepper.
- When the grill is ready, dip a clean tea towel in the vegetable oil and wipe the grill surface with the oil.
- Place the sardines on the grill and grill them for 2–3 minutes on each side.

- Drizzle the sardines with remaining olive oil and lemon juice. Sprinkle them with the oregano and serve.

GRILLED WHOLE FISH

Serves 4

- 4 (1/2-pound) whole fish (sea bream or red snapper), cleaned, gutted, and scaled 1/2 cup extra-virgin olive oil 4 teaspoons salt
- 1 1/2 teaspoons pepper 1 large lemon, thinly sliced
- 2 tablespoons chopped fresh oregano
- 2 tablespoons fresh thyme leaves
- 2 tablespoons chopped fresh rosemary
- 2 tablespoons chopped fresh tarragon
- 3 tablespoons vegetable oil
- 1/2 cup Ladolemono

Directions

- Rinse the fish and pat them dry with a paper towel. Rub the fish on both sides with the olive oil. Then sprinkle both sides and the cavity with the salt and pepper. Refrigerate the fish for 30 minutes and then return them to room temperature. Fill the cavity of each fish with equal amounts of the lemon slices and herbs.
- Preheat a gas or charcoal grill to medium-high. Brush the grill surface to make sure it is thoroughly clean. When the grill is ready, dip a clean tea towel in the vegetable oil and wipe the grill surface with the oil.

- Place the fish on the grill and grill for 5–6 minutes per side.
- Serve the fish with Ladolemono sauce. Serve immediately.

OLIVE OIL–POACHED COD

Serves 4

- 4 (6-ounce) fresh cod fillets, skins removed
- 2½–3 cups extra-virgin olive oil 1 teaspoon salt
- 2 tablespoons fresh lemon juice
- 1 tablespoon grated lemon zest

Directions

- Rinse the fillets and pat them dry with a paper towel.
- Choose a pot that will just fit the fillets and fill it with the oil. Bring the oil to a temperature of 210°F. Adjust the heat to keep the temperature at 210°F while poaching the fish.
- Carefully place the fillets in the oil and poach them for 6 minutes or until the fish is opaque in color. Carefully remove the fish from the oil and put it on a plate. Sprinkle the fish with salt.
- Spoon some of the warm oil over the fish and then drizzle it with lemon juice. Sprinkle the zest over the fish and serve it immediately.

PLAKI-STYLE BAKED FISH

Serves 4

- 1 (2-pound) whole fish, cleaned, scaled, and gutted

- 2 teaspoons salt, divided
- 1¼ teaspoons pepper, divided 1½ cups chopped fresh parsley 4 medium potatoes, peeled and cut into wedges
- 2 large cubanelle peppers, stemmed, seeded, and sliced 5 cloves garlic, peeled and roughly chopped
- 2 large tomatoes (1 diced and 1 halved and sliced), divided 4 tablespoons chopped fresh oregano or 2 teaspoons dried oregano ½ cup extra-virgin olive oil 5 tablespoons flour
- 1 teaspoon sweet paprika
- 1 cup hot water

Directions

- Preheat the oven to 350°F. Rinse the fish and pat it dry with a paper towel. Season the fish on both sides and in the cavity with 1½ teaspoons of salt and ¾ teaspoon of pepper.
- Sprinkle the parsley on the bottom of a large baking dish. Top the parsley with the potatoes, peppers, garlic, tomatoes, and oregano. Place the fish on top of the vegetables.
- In a medium bowl, whisk the oil, flour, and paprika. Pour the oil mixture over the fish. Pour the hot water over the surrounding vegetables. Season with the remaining salt and pepper.
- Bake on the middle rack of the oven for 40–45 minutes.
- Serve the fish over a bed of the vegetables. Spoon some of the sauce over the fish. Serve immediately.

PISTACHIO-CRUSTED HALIBUT

Serves 4

- 1/2 cup shelled unsalted pistachios, roughly chopped 2 teaspoons grated lemon zest
- 1 teaspoon grated lime zest
- 2 teaspoons grated orange zest
- 4 teaspoons chopped fresh parsley
- 1 cup bread crumbs
- 1/4 cup extra-virgin olive oil 4 (6-ounce) halibut fillets, skins removed
- 1 1/2 teaspoons salt
- 1/2 teaspoon pepper
- 4 teaspoons Dijon mustard

Directions

- Preheat the oven to 400°F. Put the pistachios, zests, parsley, and bread crumbs into the food processor and pulse to combine the ingredients. With the processor running, add the oil until it is well incorporated.
- Rinse the fish and pat it dry with a paper towel. Season the fish with the salt and pepper.
- Brush the tops of the fish with the mustard. Divide the pistachio mixture evenly and place some on the top of each fish. Press down on the mixture to help the crust adhere.
- Line a baking sheet with parchment paper and carefully place the crusted fish on the baking sheet. Bake it in the upper middle rack of the oven for 20 minutes or until the crust is golden brown.
- Let the fish cool for 5 minutes, and serve it immediately.

ROASTED SEA BASS WITH POTATOES AND FENNEL

Serves 2

- 4 medium potatoes, peeled and halved
- 1 small onion, peeled and sliced
- 2 tablespoons chopped fresh parsley
- 1 cup thinly sliced fennel
- 1 1/2 teaspoons grated lemon zest
- 1 tablespoon fresh lemon juice
- 1/3 cup plus 2 tablespoons extra-virgin olive oil, divided 2 teaspoons salt, divided
- 1 teaspoon pepper, divided
- 1/2 cup Basic Vegetable Stock
- 2 ripe medium tomatoes, sliced
- 2 (1/2-pound) whole European sea bass, cleaned, gutted, and scaled
- 6 tablespoons chopped fennel fronds, divided
- 4 scallions, softened in boiling water for 10 seconds 8 kalamata olives, pitted
- 4 caper berries, rinsed
- 1/4 cup dry white wine
- 1 large lemon, cut into wedges

Directions

- Preheat the oven to 450°F. Place the potatoes, onions, parsley, fennel, lemon zest, and lemon juice in a medium baking dish. Add 1/3 cup of oil and toss to combine the ingredients. Season with 1 teaspoon of salt and 1⁄2 teaspoon of pepper. Stir in the stock.

- Top the potatoes and fennel with the tomatoes. Bake in the middle rack of the oven for 25 minutes.

- In the meantime, rinse the fish and pat it dry with a paper towel. Rub both sides of each fish with the remaining oil, and then season both sides and the cavity with the remaining salt and pepper. Place 2 tablespoons of fennel fronds in each cavity. Wrap 2 scallions around each fish.

- Take the baking dish out of the oven; place the fish on top of the vegetables. Sprinkle with the olives and caper berries. Pour the wine over the fish and vegetables. Bake the dish on the middle rack of the oven for 20–25 minutes or until the potatoes are tender and the fish is golden.

- Place each fish over a bed of the cooked vegetables. Garnish with the remaining fennel fronds and serve with the lemon wedges.

RED MULLET SAVORO STYLE

Serves 4

- 4 (1⁄2-pound) whole red mullet, cleaned, gutted, and scaled 2 teaspoons salt
- 1 cup all-purpose flour
- 2⁄3 cup extra-virgin olive oil, divided 6 or 7 sprigs fresh rosemary
- 8 cloves garlic, peeled and coarsely chopped

- 2⁄3 cup red wine vinegar

Directions

- Rinse the fish and pat them dry with a paper towel. Season both sides and the cavity of the fish with salt. Let them sit for 20 minutes. Dredge the fish in flour and set aside.

- Heat 1⁄3 cup of oil in a frying pan over medium-high heat for 1 minute or until the oil is hot. Fry the fish (in batches) for 4–5 minutes a side or until golden. Place the fish on a serving platter. Discard the frying oil and wipe the pan clean.

- Add the remaining oil to the pan and heat for 1 minute. Add the rosemary; fry until it crisps and turns an olive color. Remove the rosemary from the oil. Stir the garlic into the oil and keep stirring until the garlic turns golden. Immediately add the vinegar. Stir until the sauce has thickened and becomes a little sweet.

- Pour the sauce over the fish and serve immediately. Garnish the fish with the fried rosemary.

SPINACH-STUFFED SOLE

Serves 4

- 1⁄4 cup extra-virgin olive oil, divided 4 scallions, ends trimmed and sliced
- 1 pound package frozen spinach, thawed and drained
- 3 tablespoons chopped fennel fronds, or tarragon
- 1 teaspoon salt, divided

- 1/2 teaspoon pepper, divided 4 (6-ounce) sole fillets, skins removed
- 2 tablespoons plus
- 1 1/2 teaspoons grated lemon zest, divided
- 1 teaspoon sweet paprika

Directions

- Preheat the oven to 400°F. Heat 2 tablespoons of oil in a medium skillet over medium heat for 30 seconds. Add the scallions and cook them for 3–4 minutes. Allow the scallions to cool to room temperature.
- In a bowl, combine the scallions, spinach, and fennel. Season the ingredients with 1/2 teaspoon of salt and 1/4 teaspoon of pepper.
- Rinse the fish fillets and pat them dry with a paper towel. Rub the fish with the remaining oil and sprinkle them with 2 tablespoons of lemon zest. Season the fillets with remaining salt and pepper, and sprinkle them with the paprika.
- Divide the spinach filling among the fillets; to ensure that the fillets don't unravel when baking, place the stuffing on the skin side. Roll up each fillet, starting from the widest end. Use two toothpicks to secure each fillet. Place the fillets on a baking sheet lined with parchment paper, and drizzle the remaining oil over them.
- Bake on the middle rack of the oven for 15–20 minutes. Remove the toothpicks and sprinkle the fillets with the remaining lemon zest. Serve immediately.

GRILLED OCTOPUS

Serves 4

- 2 1/2- to 3-pound octopus, cleaned and beak removed 3 bay leaves
- 1/4 cup red wine 3 tablespoons balsamic vinegar, divided
- 2/3 cup extra-virgin olive oil, divided 1 teaspoon dried oregano
- 1 teaspoon salt
- 1 teaspoon pepper
- 1 large lemon, cut into wedges

Directions

- Put the octopus and bay leaves in a large pot over medium-high heat. Cover the pot and cook the octopus for 5–8 minutes. Uncover the pot to see whether the octopus has released some liquid (about a cup). If the octopus hasn't released its liquid, just cover and continue cooking for another 5 minutes or until it has released its liquid. Reduce the heat to medium-low and cook for 45 minutes or until the octopus is tender.
- Add the wine and 2 tablespoons of vinegar. Remove the pot from the heat and allow the octopus to cool to room temperature in the liquid.
- Preheat a gas or charcoal grill to medium-high. Remove the octopus from the liquid and cut it into pieces, leaving each tentacle whole. In a large bowl, combine the octopus, 1/3 cup of oil, the oregano, and the remaining vinegar. Season it with the salt and pepper.

- Place the octopus on the grill and cook for 2–3 minutes a side.
- Drizzle the grilled octopus with the remaining oil and serve it with the lemon wedges.

SCALLOPS SAGANAKI

Serves 4

- 16 medium scallops, rinsed and patted dry
- 1 teaspoon salt
- 1/2 teaspoon pepper 1/2 cup extra-virgin olive oil 1/3 cup dry white wine
- 2 ounces ouzo
- 2 tablespoons fresh lemon juice
- 6 cloves garlic, peeled and thinly sliced
- 1 small red chili pepper, stemmed and thinly sliced
- 1/2 teaspoon sweet paprika 1 small leek, ends trimmed, thoroughly cleaned, cut lengthwise, and julienned into matchsticks 2/3 cup bread crumbs 2 tablespoons chopped fresh parsley
- 1 large lemon, cut into wedges

Directions

- Preheat the oven to 450°F. Season both sides of the scallops with the salt and pepper. Place the scallops in a medium baking dish (or divide them among four small baking dishes or ramekins). Set aside.
- In a medium bowl, whisk the oil, wine, ouzo, lemon juice, garlic, chili, and sweet paprika. Pour the sauce over the scallops; top with the leeks and then the bread crumbs.
- Bake on the middle rack for 8–10 minutes. Set the oven to broil and bake for another 2–3 minutes or until the bread crumbs are golden.
- Let the scallops cool for 5 minutes and top them with parsley. Serve the scallops with the lemon wedges.

GRILLED GROUPER STEAKS

Serves 4

- 1/4 cup extra-virgin olive oil
- 1 tablespoon grated lemon zest
- 1/2 cup dry white wine 1/2 teaspoon chopped fresh rosemary 4 (1/2-pound) grouper steaks, rinsed and dried 3 tablespoons vegetable oil
- 1 1/2 teaspoons salt

Directions

- In a medium baking dish, whisk the oil, zest, wine, and rosemary. Add the fish and toss. Cover with plastic and refrigerate for 1 hour. Allow the fish to return to room temperature for 30 minutes before grilling.
- Preheat a gas or charcoal grill to medium-high. Dip a clean tea towel in the vegetable oil and wipe the grill surface with the oil.
- Season the fish on both sides with the salt. Place fish on the grill and grill for 5–6 minutes per side. Serve.

GRILLED CALAMARI

Serves 4

- 4 (5-inch-long) squid, cleaned
- 1⁄4 cup extra-virgin olive oil 1 clove garlic, peeled and minced
- 1 teaspoon salt
- 1⁄2 teaspoon pepper
- 3 tablespoons vegetable oil
- 2 tablespoons fresh lemon juice
- 1⁄2 teaspoon dried oregano

Directions

- Preheat a gas or charcoal grill to medium-high heat. In a medium bowl, combine the squid, olive oil, garlic, salt, and pepper.
- Dip a clean tea towel in the vegetable oil and wipe the grill surface with the oil. Place the squid on the grill and cook for 2–3 minutes per side.
- Drizzle lemon juice on the squid, sprinkle it with oregano, and serve it warm.

GRILLED LOBSTER

Serves 4

- 4 (1⁄4–1⁄2 pound) live lobsters, split lengthwise 2⁄3 cup plus 1⁄4 cup extra-virgin olive oil, divided 1⁄2 teaspoons salt, divided 1⁄2 teaspoon pepper 3⁄4 teaspoon sweet paprika 1 clove garlic, peeled and minced
- 2 tablespoons fresh lemon juice
- 1⁄2 tablespoons Dijon mustard 1 scallion, ends trimmed and finely chopped

- 1 tablespoon chopped fresh parsley
- 1 tablespoon dried oregano
- 3 tablespoons vegetable oil

Directions

- Preheat a gas or charcoal grill to medium-high. Brush the grill surface to make sure it is thoroughly clean. Brush the flesh side of the lobster with
- 1⁄4 cup olive oil and season it with 1 teaspoon of salt, pepper, and paprika. Break off the claws and reserve them.
- In a medium bowl, whisk the remaining oil, garlic, lemon juice, mustard, scallion, parsley, oregano, and remaining salt. Set the sauce aside.
- When the grill is ready (medium-high heat), dip a clean tea towel in the vegetable oil and wipe the grill surface with the oil.
- Place the lobster claws on the grill first because they need longer to grill. A minute later, place the lobster bodies on the grill, flesh-side down.
- Grill for 3–4 minutes and then flip the bodies and claws. Grill for another 2–3 minutes or until the shells have turned red and the meat is cooked.
- Drizzle the sauce over the lobsters and serve the remaining sauce on the side.

GRILLED JUMBO SHRIMP

Serves 4

- 1⁄4 cup extra-virgin olive oil
- 3⁄4 teaspoon salt
- 1⁄4 teaspoon pepper

- 1/2 teaspoon sweet paprika
- 12 large jumbo shrimp, deveined but shells on
- 1/2 cup butter
- 2 tablespoons fresh lemon juice
- 1 clove garlic, peeled and minced
- 1/8 teaspoon red pepper flakes
- 1 teaspoon minced fresh ginger
- 1 tablespoon chopped fresh parsley
- 1 tablespoon chopped fresh chives
- 3 tablespoons vegetable oil

Directions

- Preheat a gas or charcoal grill to medium-high. Brush the grill surface to make sure it is thoroughly clean. In a medium bowl, whisk together olive oil, salt, pepper, and paprika. Add the shrimp and marinate for 10 minutes.
- In a small pot over medium heat, cook the butter, lemon juice, garlic, red pepper flakes, and ginger until the butter melts. Add the parsley and chives. Keep the sauce warm.
- When the grill is ready (medium-high heat), dip a clean tea towel in the vegetable oil and wipe the grill surface with the oil. Place the shrimp on the grill and grill for 2 minutes per side or until they turn pink.
- Drizzle the shrimp with the butter sauce and serve the remaining sauce on the side.

OCTOPUS STIFADO

Serves 4

- 1 (2-pound) octopus, cleaned and beak removed
- 1/2 cup extra-virgin olive oil 1 1/2 cups pearl onions, blanched and skins removed 1/2 cup dry white wine 1/4 cup red wine vinegar 2 tablespoons tomato paste
- 3 bay leaves
- 6 or 7 whole allspice berries
- 1/2 teaspoon grated orange zest 1 teaspoon salt
- 1/2 teaspoon pepper
- 1/8 teaspoon ground cinnamon
- 1/3 cup chopped fresh dill

Directions

- Put the octopus in a large oven-safe pot over medium-high heat, cover the pot, and cook for 10 minutes. Take the pot off the heat, remove the octopus from the liquid, reserve the liquid, and let the octopus cool.
- Preheat the oven to 350°F. To the pot with the reserved octopus cooking liquid, add the oil, onions, wine, vinegar, tomato paste, bay leaves, allspice, and zest. Season the sauce with salt and pepper.
- Cut up the octopus; separate the tentacles from the head and roughly chop up the head. Return the octopus to the pot, and cover it.
- Bake the octopus in the oven on the middle rack for 90 minutes or until the octopus is fork-tender. Uncover it, and bake for another 10 minutes to thicken the sauce.

- Remove the bay leaves, and stir in the cinnamon and dill. Serve the octopus hot.

OYSTERS ON THE HALF SHELL

Serves 4

- 16 live fresh oysters
- 4 cups crushed ice
- 1 large lemon, cut into wedges

Directions

- Place an oyster on a steady work surface with the hinged end facing up. Using a tea towel to help you hold the oyster, grip it with one hand. With the other hand, carefully stick a knife or oyster shucker into the hinge. Dig the knife into the hinge, wiggling the knife until the shell begins to open.
- Slide the knife across the top shell to disconnect the muscle from the shell.
- You should be able to open the oyster. Discard the top shell. Slip the knife underneath the oyster and disconnect it from the bottom shell. Remove any pieces of dirt or broken shell. Smell the oyster; it should smell like the sea. If it doesn't, discard it.
- Repeat this process with the remaining oysters.
- Serve the oysters (in their bottom shells) on a bed of crushed ice with the lemon wedges.

COD WITH RAISINS

Serves 4

- 1 1/2 pounds salted cod, fresh or frozen 3–4 tablespoons extra-virgin olive oil
- 2 cooking onions, chopped, but not too finely
- 1 tablespoon tomato paste, diluted in 3/4 cup water
- 3/4 cup black raisins
- 1 cup water

Directions

- If using salted cod, make sure to soak in water at least 24 hours, changing water several times to remove salt.
- Heat olive oil in a cooking pot over medium heat. Add onions; sauté lightly for a few minutes. Make sure to stir constantly to avoid browning the onion; it should be tender but not burned.
- Add tomato paste to onions; bring to boil and simmer for 10 minutes.
- Add raisins and continue to cook for 3 more minutes.
- Add water; bring to boil and simmer for 30 minutes, until raisins have expanded.
- Add cod; simmer for 15 minutes, until the sauce has reduced. Serve with raisin-onion sauce spooned over top.

AEGEAN BAKED SOLE

Serves 4

- 8 sole fillets
- Salt and pepper to taste
- 2 lemons
- 4 tablespoons extra-virgin olive oil, divided
- 1 teaspoon dried oregano

- 1⁄4 cup capers
- 4 tablespoons chopped fresh dill
- 2 tablespoons chopped fresh green onion (or celery leaves or parsley)

Directions

- Preheat the oven to 250°F.
- Wash fish well under cold water and pat dry with a paper towel. Season fillets with salt and pepper and set aside.
- Slice 1 lemon into thin slices, then cut slices in half.
- Pour 2 tablespoons olive oil into a baking dish; layer fish and lemon slices alternately.
- Sprinkle oregano, capers, dill, and onion over fish and lemon slices.
- Drizzle remaining olive oil and squeeze juice of remaining lemon over everything.
- Cover and bake for 30 minutes.

BAKED SEA BREAM WITH FETA AND TOMATO

Serves 4

- 4 small whole sea bream
- 1⁄2 cup extra-virgin olive oil 6 ripe tomatoes, peeled and minced
- 1 teaspoon dried marjoram
- Salt and pepper
- 1⁄2 cup water
- 1⁄2 cup fresh parsley, finely chopped
- 1⁄2 pound Greek feta cheese

Directions

- Preheat the oven to 400°F.

- Wash and clean fish well; set aside to drain.
- In a saucepan, heat olive oil; add tomatoes, marjoram, salt, pepper, and water. Bring to a boil; simmer for 15 minutes.
- Place fish side by side in the baking dish; pour sauce over top and sprinkle with parsley. Bake for 30 minutes.
- Crumble feta cheese; remove baking dish from oven and sprinkle feta over fish. Return to oven to bake for another 5–7 minutes, until cheese starts to melt. Remove and serve immediately.

BAKED TUNA

Serves 4

- 4 center-cut tuna fillets, 6–8 ounces each (2 pounds total) 1⁄4 cup extra-virgin olive oil, divided 1 large yellow onion, sliced
- 1 large green pepper, diced
- 2 cloves garlic, minced or pressed
- 2 tablespoons chopped parsley
- 1 teaspoon dried marjoram (or 1⁄2 teaspoon dried oregano)
- Salt and fresh-ground pepper to taste
- 2 cups peeled tomatoes, finely minced (canned tomatoes are fine)
- 1⁄2 cup water

Directions

- Preheat the oven to 400°F.
- Wash tuna steaks well and set aside.
- In a large frying pan, heat 2 tablespoons olive oil on medium-high. Sauté onion and green pepper until soft.

- Add garlic, parsley, marjoram, salt, and pepper; stir over heat for another minute or so.
- Add tomatoes and water; bring to a boil. Lower heat to medium-low and simmer for 15–20 minutes.
- Place tuna steaks in a baking dish along with the remaining olive oil, making sure to coat the tuna with the oil; pour the sauce over the top.
- Bake uncovered for 45 minutes. Serve immediately, spooning some sauce over each portion.

BRAISED CUTTLEFISH

Serves 4–6

- 2 pounds cuttlefish, cleaned and cut into strips
- 1/3 cup extra-virgin olive oil 2 large onions, diced
- 3 cloves garlic, pressed or finely chopped
- 1 cup red wine
- 2 cups minced tomatoes
- 2 tablespoons fresh parsley, finely chopped
- 1 teaspoon dried marjoram
- 1 bay leaf
- Salt and pepper to taste

Directions

- Clean cuttlefish and cut into strips; set aside to drain well. Make sure to pat strips dry with a paper towel before using in order to avoid hot oil pops.

- Heat olive oil in a pan; sauté onions until soft.
- Add garlic and sauté for another 30 seconds or so before adding (drained) cuttlefish. Continue to sauté and stir continuously until cuttlefish starts to turn a yellowish color, approximately 6–8 minutes.
- Add wine and continue to cook for another 10 minutes, stirring regularly.
- Add tomatoes, parsley, marjoram, bay leaf, salt, and pepper; cover and simmer over medium-low heat for approximately 90 minutes, until sauce has thickened and cuttlefish is tender. Add 1/2–1 cup water to pan should liquid thicken before cuttlefish has softened sufficiently.
- Serve warm with fresh bread.

STOVETOP FISH

Serves 4

- 2 pounds whitefish fillets
- 3 tablespoons extra-virgin olive oil
- 4 or 5 cloves garlic, minced
- 1 pound ripe tomatoes, peeled and minced 6–8 fresh mint leaves, finely chopped Salt and pepper
- 1 tablespoon dried oregano
- 1/2 cup water 1 small bunch fresh parsley

Directions

- Wash fish fillets and pat with a paper towel to dry.
- Heat olive oil in a large frying pan and quickly sauté the garlic.

- Add the tomatoes, mint, salt, pepper, and oregano. Bring to a boil and let simmer for 10 minutes, until thickened.
- Add the water and continue to simmer for another 3–4 minutes.
- Place the fish in the pan and allow to simmer for 15 minutes. Do not stir; simply shake pan gently from time to time to avoid sticking.
- Garnish with chopped parsley and serve immediately with rice.

GRILLED SEA BASS

Serves 4

- 4 whole sea bass (1 1/2 pounds each), gutted and scaled Salt and pepper
- 4 lemons
- 1/4 cup extra-virgin olive oil
- 1 teaspoon dried oregano
- 1 cup fresh parsley, finely chopped

Directions

- Wash the fish well inside and out. Using a sharp knife, cut several diagonal slits on both sides of each fish. Sprinkle with salt and pepper, including inside cavity, and set aside.
- Squeeze juice from 2 lemons and mix with olive oil and oregano.
- Slice remaining 2 lemons into thin slices and stuff each fish with chopped parsley and several lemon slices.
- Brush both sides of each fish liberally with olive oil and lemon mixture and set aside for 10 minutes.

- Heat grill to medium heat; brush grilling rack with oil. Place fish on hot rack and close grill cover.
- Cook for 15 minutes, until fish flakes easily. Brush with remaining olive oil and lemon mixture and serve hot.

OCTOPUS IN WINE

Serves 4

- 1 large octopus
- 1 tablespoon white vinegar
- 1/2 cup extra-virgin olive oil
- 3 onions, sliced
- 4 tomatoes, diced and sieved (fresh or canned)
- 1 cup white wine
- 2 bay leaves
- 1 teaspoon whole peppercorns
- Salt and pepper
- 1/2 cup drained capers
- 1/4 cup water

Directions

- Place octopus in a saucepan with vinegar; cover and simmer over low heat until soft, approximately 15–20 minutes. Remove and cut into small pieces.
- Heat olive oil in a frying pan and sauté onions until soft.
- Add tomatoes, wine, bay leaves, peppercorns, salt, and pepper; simmer for 15 minutes.
- Add octopus, capers, and water; simmer until sauce has thickened. Remove the bay leaves; serve hot.

CIOPPINO

Serves 6

- clams
- mussels
- ounces skinless, boneless cod fillet
- 1 shallot
- 1 yellow onion
- 2 cloves garlic
- 2 stalks celery
- 2 carrots
- 3 plum tomatoes
- 1 cup dry white wine
- 3 cups Fish Stock
- 1/2 teaspoon saffron threads
- 1/4 teaspoon dried red pepper flakes
- 1/2 teaspoon extra-virgin olive oil
- 1/4 teaspoon capers

Directions

- Rinse the clams in ice-cold water. Thoroughly clean the mussels. Cut the cod into chunks. Small-dice the shallot, onion, garlic, and celery. Peel and small-dice the carrots and tomatoes (see Tomato Fritters recipe in Chapter 4 for tomato peeling instructions).
- Place the cod, vegetables, wine, stock, saffron, and pepper flakes into a large stockpot; simmer over medium heat for approximately 1 hour.
- Add the shellfish and cook until the shells open. (Discard any clams or mussels that do not open!)
- Ladle the Cioppino into bowls. Drizzle with the oil and sprinkle with the

STEAMED SNOW CRAB LEGS

Serves 6

- 6 snow crab claw clusters
- 2 pounds parsnips
- 6 celery stalks
- 1 yellow onion
- 1/2 bunch fresh parsley
- 1/2 cup white wine (Pinot Grigio or Sauvignon Blanc) Juice of 1 lemon
- 1 cup Fish Stock
- 3 bay leaves Fresh-cracked black pepper, to taste

Directions

- Clean the crab legs thoroughly in ice-cold water. Peel and roughly chop the parsnips. Roughly chop the celery and onion. Chop the parsley.
- Combine all the ingredients except the snow crab in a medium-size saucepot and bring to a boil; reduce to a simmer and cook uncovered for approximately 20–30 minutes.
- Add the crab legs, and cook for 10–15 minutes, until the crab is cooked. Remove the bay leaves, then serve.

STEAMED SEAFOOD DINNER

Serves 6

- 1 pound lobster
- 1/2 dozen clams 1/2 dozen oysters
- 1/2 dozen mussels
- 1/2 dozen large shrimp 1/2 dozen sea scallops 3 large potatoes
- 1/2 dozen carrots 1/2 bunch fresh parsley

- 1/2 dozen celery stalks 6 shallots
- 6 small sprigs thyme
- 1/2 cup white wine (Pinot Grigio or Sauvignon Blanc) Juice of 1 lemon
- 1 cup Seafood Stock
- 3 bay leaves
- 1/2 teaspoon Old Bay Seasoning Fresh-cracked black pepper, to taste

Directions

- Clean the shellfish thoroughly in ice-cold water. Cut the potatoes in half. Peel the carrots (leave whole). Chop the parsley. (Leave the celery and shallots whole.)
- In a medium-size saucepot, bring the wine, lemon juice, and stock to a boil. Add the potatoes, carrots, celery, shallots, herbs, and spices; let simmer for 45 minutes. Add the rest of the ingredients and reduce to a simmer; cook for 10–15 more minutes. Remove the thyme sprigs, then serve.

GRILLED FISH WITH POLENTA

Serves 6

- 1/2 serrano chili pepper 2 teaspoons olive oil
- 1 quart Fish Stock
- 1 1/2 cups cornmeal 1 teaspoon extra-virgin olive oil
- 1 1/2 pounds red snapper Pinch of coarse sea salt Fresh-cracked black pepper, to taste
- 3 ounces manchego cheese
- 1 tablespoon cider vinegar

Directions

- Preheat grill to medium heat. Stem, seed, and dice the serrano chili pepper.
- Heat the olive oil in a stockpot over medium heat. Lightly sauté the chili, then add the stock and bring to a boil.
- Whisk in the cornmeal slowly; cook for approximately 20–30 minutes, stirring frequently (add more broth if necessary).
- While the polenta cooks, lightly dip the fish in the extra-virgin olive oil and place on a rack to drain. Season with salt and pepper.
- When the polenta is done cooking, remove it from the heat and add the manchego; keep warm.
- Grill the fish for 3–5 minutes on each side, depending on the thickness of the fish.
- To serve, spoon out a generous dollop of polenta on each serving plate and arrange the fish on top. Drizzle with the vinegar.

BACCALÁ

Serves 6

- 1 1/2 pounds baccalá (salted cod) 3 cloves garlic
- 2 plum tomatoes
- 1 stalk celery
- 1/2 bunch fresh parsley
- 1 tablespoon olive oil
- 1/4 cup dry white wine
- 1/2 cup Fish Stock
- Fresh-cracked black pepper, to taste

Directions

- Soak the baccalá for 24 hours in water.
- Mince the garlic. Medium-dice the tomatoes and celery. Mince the parsley.
- Heat the oil in a large sauté pan over medium-high heat. Add the baccalá, garlic, tomatoes, and celery; sauté the baccalá on each side for approximately 1 minute. Add the wine and let it reduce by half. Add the stock and pepper; simmer, covered, for 10 minutes.
- Serve with the cooking liquid and sprinkle with parsley.

FLOUNDER WITH BALSAMIC REDUCTION

Serves 6

- 1⁄4 cup all-purpose flour 1 tablespoon cornmeal
- 11⁄2 pounds flounder 1 tablespoon olive oil
- 1⁄2 cup Balsamic Reduction
- Fresh-cracked black pepper, to taste
- 3 sprigs dill

Directions

- Mix together the flour and cornmeal; coat the flounder in the mixture.
- Heat the oil over medium heat in a large sauté pan. Cook the flounder for approximately 7 minutes on each side.
- While the flounder cooks, heat the Balsamic Reduction sauce. Serve the fish drizzled with the sauce and sprinkled with pepper; garnish each serving with half a sprig of dill.

HALIBUT ROULADE

Serves 6

- 1-pound halibut fillet
- 1⁄2 pound shrimp 3 limes
- 1⁄4 bunch cilantro 3 cloves garlic
- 1⁄2 leek 1 tablespoon olive oil
- Fresh-cracked black pepper, to taste
- 1 cup seafood Demi-Glace Reduction Sauce

Directions

- Soak 12 wooden skewers in water for at least 2 hours.
- Preheat grill.
- Clean the halibut and keep chilled. Completely remove the shells and tails from the shrimp (save for future use in stock). Slice the shrimp in half lengthwise and remove the veins. Juice 2 of the limes and grate the rinds for zest. Cut the remaining lime into 6 wedges. Reserve 6 whole leaves of cilantro for garnish and chop the rest. Mince the garlic and finely slice the leek.
- Butterfly the halibut fillet lengthwise to make a 1⁄2- to 3⁄4-inch-thick fillet. Lay the fillet out, then layer the shrimp, half of the lime zest, half of the chopped cilantro, the garlic, and leek. Gently roll up the stuffed fillet, then cut into 6 pinwheels. Insert 2 skewers into each pinwheel, forming an X, which will hold the pinwheels together. Brush with some of the oil, and grill for 4 minutes on each side.

- To serve, sprinkle each with pepper and the remaining zest and cilantro. Drizzle with the remaining oil and Demi-Glace Reduction Sauce.

PARCHMENT SALMON

Serves 6

- 1⁄4 cup Compound Butter
- 1⁄2 pound fresh forest mushrooms
- 1 tablespoon minced shallot
- 2 bunches green onions, chopped
- 2 teaspoons chopped fresh marjoram
- 1 1⁄2 pounds salmon fillet
- 1⁄4 cup dry white wine

Directions

- Combine the butter, mushrooms, shallot, green onions, and marjoram. Roll in parchment paper and chill for a minimum of 6 hours, until firm.
- Preheat the oven to 400°F.
- Cut the salmon into 4 portions and place each on a folded sheet of parchment paper. Top each with 2 ample slices of the butter. Sprinkle each with about 1 tablespoon of the white wine. Fold up each, folding the parchment over the top and continuing to fold until well sealed.
- Roast for 7–10 minutes, until the paper is slightly brown. Slit open paper and serve immediately.

BARBECUED MARINATED TUNA

Serves 6

- 1 1⁄2 pounds fresh tuna
- 1⁄4 cup apple juice
- 1⁄4 cup dry red wine
- 1 tablespoon olive oil
- 1⁄2 tablespoon honey
- 1⁄4 cup minced serrano chili pepper Zest of 1 lemon
- 2 anchovies, chopped
- Fresh-cracked black pepper, to taste

Directions

- Rinse the fish in ice water and pat dry.
- Blend together the juice, wine, oil, honey, chili, and zest. Pour the mixture over the tuna and let marinate for 30 minutes.
- Preheat grill.
- Place the fish on the grill (reserve the marinade) and cook for 2–4 minutes on each side, depending on the thickness of the fish and desired doneness.
- While the tuna cooks, place the marinade in a small saucepan over medium heat and reduce by half.
- To serve, plate the tuna and drizzle with marinade syrup, then sprinkle with anchovies and pepper.

FISH CHILI WITH BEANS

Serves 6

- 1 1⁄4 pounds fresh fish (sea bass, halibut, or red snapper) 1 leek
- 1 medium yellow onion
- 12 fresh plum tomatoes
- 4 ounces firm tofu
- 1 fresh jalapeño
- 1 fresh serrano
- 1 teaspoon curry powder

- 1 teaspoon chili powder
- 1⁄4 teaspoon cayenne pepper Fresh-cracked black pepper, to taste
- 2 tablespoons olive oil
- 2 cups cooked beans (pintos, cannellini, or red kidney)
- 1⁄2 cup dry red wine
- 1 cup Seafood Stock
- 1⁄2 cup brewed strong coffee 1 teaspoon brown sugar
- 1 tablespoon honey

Directions

- Rinse the fish in ice water and pat dry. Slice the leek and medium-dice the onion. Dice the tomatoes. Cut the tofu into large dice. Mince the jalapeño and serrano. Mix together the curry and chili powders, the cayenne, and black pepper.
- Heat most of the oil over medium heat in a large saucepan. Add the leeks, onions, tomatoes, and tofu; cook for 2 minutes. Sprinkle with some of the seasoning mixture, then add all the remaining ingredients except the fish; stew for approximately 60 minutes.
- Preheat grill to medium temperature.
- Brush the fish with the remaining olive oil and seasoning mixture; grill on each side until cooked through (the cooking time will vary depending on the type of fish and thickness), about 5–15 minutes.
- To serve, ladle the stew into bowls and top with grilled fish.

SAUTÉED RED SNAPPER

Serves 6

- 11⁄2 pounds fresh red snapper
- 1⁄4 teaspoon turmeric
- 1 teaspoon curry powder
- 1⁄4 teaspoon garam masala Fresh-cracked black pepper, to taste
- 1 cup all-purpose unbleached flour
- 1⁄4 cup plain nonfat yogurt
- 1⁄4 cup buttermilk
- 2 tablespoons olive oil

Directions

- Rinse the fish in ice water and pat dry. Cut the fish into 6 serving pieces. Sift together the turmeric, curry powder, garam masala, black pepper, and flour. In a separate bowl, mix together the yogurt and buttermilk.
- Dust the fish with the flour mixture, then dip into the yogurt mix, and back into the flour mixture.
- Heat the oil over medium-high heat in a large sauté pan; sauté the fish on each side until crispy, golden brown, and flaky. Drain on rack lined with paper towels and serve.

SALMON AND HADDOCK TERRINE

Serves 6

- 1 tablespoon olive oil
- 3⁄4 pound fresh salmon fillet
- 3⁄4 pound haddock fillet 3 cloves garlic
- 1 medium eggplant

- Fresh-cracked black pepper, to taste
- Kosher salt, to taste
- 1 head arugula
- 2 Roasted Red Peppers

Directions

- Preheat the oven to 375°F. Grease a loaf pan with the olive oil.
- Rinse the fish in ice water and pat dry. Thinly slice the garlic. Cut eggplant in half lengthwise; roast for 20 minutes.
- Season the fish with black pepper and salt. In the prepared pan, layer the salmon, cooled eggplant, arugula, haddock, cooled red peppers, garlic, then more arugula, and top with eggplant.
- Wrap tightly with foil and bake for 20 minutes. Unwrap and press down on the layered ingredients; rewrap tightly and bake for 10–20 minutes longer, until thoroughly cooked. Remove from oven and let cool in the refrigerator overnight.
- To serve, unmold from loaf pan. Slice and serve.

TILAPIA WITH SMOKED GOUDA

Serves 6

- 1 1⁄4 pounds fresh tilapia fillets 6 fresh plum tomatoes
- turnips
- 1 leek
- 1 shallot
- 3 cloves garlic

- 1⁄4 bunch parsley 3 ounces smoked Gouda
- 1 tablespoon olive oil
- 1 cup Fish Stock
- 1⁄4 cup dry red wine Fresh-cracked black pepper, to taste

Directions

- Preheat the oven to 375°F.
- Rinse the fish in ice water and pat dry. Medium-dice the tomatoes. Peel and thinly slice the turnips. Finely slice the leek. Mince the shallot and garlic. Chop the parsley. Grate the cheese.
- Paint a medium-size baking dish with olive oil, then layer the leek, turnips, shallot, garlic, and fish. Pour in the stock and wine; bake, covered, for 30–40 minutes.
- Uncover and sprinkle with tomatoes and cheese. Return to oven until cheese is completely melted. Serve hot, sprinkled with parsley and pepper.
- Using Wine with Fish
- Use a nice dry wine to stand up to the smoky flavor of the cheese. Generally speaking, a light, nonrobust, drinking red wine works well in fish dishes.

Grilled Salmon

Total time: 23 minutes

Prep time: 15 minutes

Cook time: 8 minutes

Yield: 4 servings

Ingredients

- 2 tbsp. freshly squeezed lemon juice

- 1 tbsp. minced garlic
- 1 tbsp. chopped fresh parsley
- 4 tbsp. chopped fresh basil
- 4 salmon fillets, each 5 ounces
- Extra virgin olive oil?
- Sea salt and cracked black pepper, to taste
- 4 green olives, chopped
- Cracked black pepper
- 4 thin slices lemon

Directions

- Lightly coat grill rack with olive oil cooking spray and position it 4 inches from heat; heat grill to medium high.
- Combine lemon juice, minced garlic, parsley and basil in a small bowl.
- Coat fish with extra virgin olive oil and season with sea salt and pepper.
- Top each fish fillet with equal amount of garlic mixture and place on the heated grill, herb-side down.
- Grill over high heat for about 4 minutes or until the edges turn white; turn over and transfer the fish to aluminum foil.
- Reduce heat and continue grilling for about 4 minutes more.
- Transfer the grilled fish to plates and garnish with lemon slices and green olives.
- Serve immediately.

MEDITERRANEAN MEAT, BEEF AND PORK RECIPES

Liver with Apple and Onion

Total time: 35 minutes

Prep time: 10 minutes

Cook time: 25 minutes

Yield: 2 servings

Ingredients

- Extra virgin olive oil spray
- ½ lb. onion
- 2 Granny Smith apples
- 1 cup water
- 1 tbsp. fresh lemon juice
- 1 tbsp. white wine vinegar
- 1 tsp. brown sugar
- 1 tbsp. fresh rosemary, plus sprigs for garnish
- 2 tbsp. dried currants
- 2 tsp. unsalted butter
- 8 ounces calves' liver
- ¼ cup white wine
- ¼ tsp. sea salt
- olive oil spray

Directions

- Preheat your oven to 200ºF.
- Spray skillet with extra virgin olive oil spray and set over medium heat; add onions and sauté for about 4 minutes or until translucent.
- Add apples and cook for about 5 minutes or until they start to brown.
- Stir in water, lemon juice, vinegar and sugar and cook until apples are tender.

- Stir in rosemary and currants, cook, stirring for about 2 minutes and divide between two plates; keep warm in the oven.
- Melt butter in the same pan until frothing.
- Stir in liver and sauté for about 10 minutes or until browned on the outside.
- Divide the liver between the two plates of apple-onion mixture.
- Add white wine to the hot pan to deglaze; cook until the liquid is reduced by half and pour equal amounts over each serving.
- Serve garnished with fresh rosemary.

Lamb Chops

Total time: 25 minutes
Prep time: 10 minutes
Cook time: 10 minutes
Standing time: 5 minutes
Yield: 4 servings
Ingredients

- 1 tbsp. dried oregano
- 1 tbsp. garlic, minced
- ¼ tsp. black pepper, freshly ground
- ½ tsp. sea salt
- 2 tbsp. lemon juice, fresh
- 8 lamb loin chops, fat trimmed off
- Cooking spray

Directions

- Preheat your broiler.
- In a small bowl, combine all the spices, herbs and lemon juice and rub this mixture on both sides of the lamb chops.

- Spray the broiler pan with the cooking spray and broil the lamb chops for 4 minutes on each side or depending on how done you want your chops. Cover the cooked lamb chops in foil and let them rest for 5 minutes and you are ready to serve.

Sage Seared Calf's Liver

Total time: 30 minutes
Prep time: 20 minutes
Cook time: 10 minutes
Yield: 4 servings
Ingredients

- 2 tsp. extra virgin olive oil
- 1 clove garlic, minced
- 8 ounces calves' liver, cut into small strips
- 1 tbsp. flat leaf parsley
- 1 tbsp. fresh sage
- 1 tsp. balsamic vinegar
- 2 tbsp. red wine
- 2 tsp. unsalted butter
- 1 tsp. fresh lemon juice
- ¼ tsp. sea salt
- Black pepper

Directions

- Heat extra virgin olive oil in a nonstick skillet set over medium heat; stir in minced garlic and sauté for about 3 minutes or until translucent and fragrant.
- Add strips of liver, parsley and sage and cook for about 5 minutes or until the meat is seared on outside.

- Transfer the liver to a warm plate and quickly deglaze the pan with vinegar, red wine, butter, and lemon juice for about 30 seconds.
- Pour the sauce over the meat and serve right away.

Seasoned Lamb Burgers

Total time: 30 minutes

Prep time: 20 minutes

Cook time: 10 minutes

Yield: 4 servings

Ingredients

- 1 ½ pounds ground lamb
- 1 tsp. ground cumin
- ½ tsp. ground cinnamon
- 1 tsp. ground ginger
- ¼ cup extra virgin olive oil, divided
- 1 tsp. black pepper, freshly ground; divided
- ¼ cup fresh cilantro
- 2 tbsp. fresh oregano
- 1 small clove garlic, pressed
- ¾ tsp. red pepper flakes, crushed
- ¼ cup fresh flat leaf parsley
- 1 tbsp. sherry vinegar
- 2 pitas, warmed and halved
- Sliced tomato
- 1 8 oz of package plain Greek yogurt

Directions

- Prepare a charcoal or gas grill fire.
- Mix the ground lamb with cumin, cinnamon, ginger, 1 tablespoon extra virgin olive oil and ½ teaspoon black pepper.

- Mix well and divide this into four burgers.
- Spray the grill with some olive oil and grill the burgers for 5 minutes on each side.
- Combine the rest of the olive oil, cilantro, oregano, garlic, red pepper flakes, parsley and vinegar in a food processor until it forms a thick paste. Serve each burger in pita bread on a plate with sliced tomato, the processed sauce and a serving of yogurt.

London Broil with Bourbon-Sautéed Mushrooms

Total time: 1 hour, 15 minutes

Prep time: 15 minutes

Cook time: 60 minutes

Yield: 3 servings

Ingredients

- ½ tsp. extra virgin olive oil
- ½ cup minced shallot
- ¾ lb. halved crimini mushrooms
- 6 tbsp. non-fat beef stock
- 3 tbsp. bourbon
- ½ tbsp. unsalted butter
- 1 tbsp. pure maple syrup
- Black pepper, to taste
- 1 lb. lean London broil
- ⅛ tsp. sea salt

Directions

- Preheat your oven to 400°F.
- Heat a nonstick skillet in oven for about 10 minutes.
- Remove and add extra virgin olive oil; swirl to coat the pan.

- Stir in shallots and mushrooms until well blended; return to oven and roast the mushrooms for about 15 minutes, stirring once with a wooden spatula.
- Stir in beef stock, bourbon, butter, maple syrup and pepper; toss and return the pan to oven; cook for 10 minutes more or until liquid is reduced by half.
- Remove pan from oven and set aside.
- Place another nonstick skillet in the oven and heat for about 10 minutes.
- In the meantime, sprinkle salt and ground pepper over the steak and place it in the hot pan.
- Roast in the oven for about 14 minutes, turning once.
- Remove the meat from oven and warm the mushrooms.
- Place steak on a cutting board and let rest for about 5 minutes.
- Thinly slice beef and serve top with sautéed mushrooms to serve.

Grilled Sage Lamb Kabob

Total time: 4 hours, 50 minutes

Marinating time: 4 hours

Prep time: 20 minutes

Cook time: 30 minutes

Yield: 2 servings

Ingredients

- 1 tbsp. fresh lemon juice
- 2 tbsp. fresh chives
- 2 tbsp. fresh flat leaf parsley
- 2 tbsp. fresh sage
- 1 tbsp. dark brown sugar
- 1 tbsp. extra virgin olive oil
- 2 tbsp. dry sherry
- 1 tbsp. pure maple syrup
- ¼ tsp. sea salt
- 8 ounces lean lamb shoulder
- 2 cups water
- 4 medium red potatoes
- White onion, cut into halves
- 6 shitake mushroom caps
- ½ red bell pepper

Directions

- In a blender, combine together lemon juice, chives, parsley, sage, brown sugar, extra virgin olive oil, sherry, maple syrup, and salt; puree until very smooth.
- Cut lamb into 8 cubes and add to a zipper bag along with the marinade; marinate in the refrigerator for at least 4 hours.
- Bring a pot with water to a rolling boil.
- Cut potatoes in halves and add to the pot along with half onion; steam for about 15 minutes. Remove from heat and let cool.
- Chop the remaining onion and pepper.
- On a skewer, alternate lamb cube, mushroom cap, pepper, onion and potato.
- Reserve the marinade.
- Grill the kabobs over hot grill, turning every 3 minutes and basting with the reserved marinade.

Lemony Pork With Lentils

Total time: 45 minutes

Prep time: 15 minutes

Cook time: 30 minutes

Chill time: 8 hours

Yield: 4 servings

Ingredients

- 2 tbsp. extra virgin olive oil, divided
- 4 (4 ounce) pork chops
- 2 tbsp. fresh lemon juice
- 1 tsp. lemon zest
- 1 clove garlic
- 2 tbsp. fresh rosemary
- 1 tbsp. parsley
- 1 tbsp. pure maple syrup
- 6 cups water, divided
- ½ cup green lentils
- 1 shallot
- 1 rib celery
- ½ cup dry sherry, divided
- 1 tsp. sea salt
- 1 tsp. unsalted butter
- ¼ tsp. red pepper flakes

Directions

- In a zipper bag, combine extra virgin olive oil, pork chops, lemon juice, lemon zest, garlic clove, rosemary, parsley, and maple syrup; refrigerate for at least 8 hours.
- Combine 3 cups of water and green lentils in a saucepan set over medium heat and cook for about 20 minutes or until lentils are just tender; drain and rinse.
- Preheat your oven to 350ºF.
- Heat a nonstick skillet over medium high heat and add the marinade; sear pork for

about 2 minutes per side and transfer the skillet to the oven.

- In the meantime, heat 1 teaspoon of extra virgin olive oil to a second nonstick skillet set over medium high heat; add shallot, red pepper flakes and celery and lower heat to medium; cook for about 4 minutes or until tender. Stir in lentils until warmed through.
- Add ¼ teaspoon sea salt and ¼ cup sherry and cook for about 2 minutes or until liquid is reduced by half. Stir in butter until melted.
- Divide the lentil mixture among four plates and top each serving with one pork chop from first skillet.
- Remove and discard garlic from marinade in the first skillet and deglaze the pan with ¼ cup sherry; increase heat and stir in ¼ teaspoon sea salt; cook until the liquid is reduced by half.
- Evenly pour the sauce over each serving and serve.

Cumin Pork Chops

Total time: 30 minutes

Prep time: 10 minutes

Cook time: 20 minutes

Yield: 1 serving

Ingredients

- 4-ounce lean center-cut pork chop
- ⅛ tsp. sea salt
- ⅛ tsp. ground cumin
- Olive oil spray
- 2 tbsp. mashed avocado
- 2 tsp. fresh cilantro leaves

Directions

- Preheat your oven to 400°F.
- Heat a large skillet over medium heat.
- In the meantime, season pork chop with sea salt and cumin.
- Spray the pan with extra virgin olive oil and add the seasoned pork chop.
- Place the pan in oven and cook for about 10 minutes, turn the pork chop over and spread the seared part with avocado.
- Return to oven and cook for about 10 minutes more or until pork is done.
- Serve pork garnished with cilantro over mashed potatoes.

Healthy Lamb Burgers

Total time: 40 minutes

Prep time: 10 minutes, plus 20 minutes resting time

Cook time: 10 minutes

Yield: 4 servings

Ingredients

- 1 tbsp. extra virgin olive oil
- 1 lb. lean ground lamb
- 2 tbsp. yogurt cheese
- ⅛ tsp. ground allspice
- ½ cup cilantro leaves, chopped
- 1 small egg white
- 1 shallot, finely chopped
- 2 cloves garlic, chopped
- 2 tsp. fresh ginger, minced
- 1 red chili pepper, chopped
- ⅛ tsp. ground cumin
- 4 cardamom seeds
- ⅛ tsp. black pepper

- ¼ tsp. sea salt
- spray olive oil
- 4 whole-wheat hamburger buns

Directions

- Mix together all the ingredients except spray olive oil and buns, and refrigerate for at least 20 minutes.
- Preheat your oven to 400° F.
- Heat extra virgin olive oil in a large nonstick skillet over medium heat.
- In the meantime, form lamb mixture into 4 burgers.
- Sear burgers in prepared pan for about 1 minute; transfer the pan to the preheated oven and cook for about 5 minutes, turn burgers over and cook for about 3 minutes more.

Herb-Maple Crusted Steak

Total time: 25 minutes

Prep time: 15 minutes

Cook time: 10 minutes

Yield: 4 servings

Ingredients

- 3 tbsp. rosemary
- 3 tbsp. fresh tarragon
- 3 tbsp. chives
- 3 tbsp. chopped oregano
- 4 tbsp. parsley
- 3 tbsp. maple syrup
- 4 (4 ounce) ribeye steaks, trimmed
- ½ tsp. sea salt
- ¼ tsp. black pepper
- spray olive oil

Directions

- Preheat your oven to 450°F.
- Heat a nonstick skillet in the oven.
- In the meantime, combine the minced herbs on a plate
- Add maple syrup to a separate bowl.
- Season steak with sea salt and pepper and dip into the maple syrup; turn to coat well.
- Dip the steak into the herbs and turn to coat well. Repeat with the remaining steak.
- Remove the skillet from oven and spray with extra virgin olive oil; add steaks to the pan and turn until well seared.
- Return to oven and cook for about 4 minutes, turn and cook the other side for about 6 minutes more.

Tenderloin with Blue Cheese Butter

Total time: 30 minutes

Prep time: 15 minutes

Cook time: 15 minutes

Yield: 2 servings

Ingredients

- ⅛ tsp. black pepper
- 1 small shallot, minced
- 1 tsp. unsalted butter
- 2 tbsp. chopped parsley
- 2 tsp. blue cheese
- Extra virgin olive oil spray
- 2 4-ounce beef tenderloin filets
- ¼ tsp. sea salt

Directions

- In a blender, blend together pepper, shallot, butter, parsley and blue cheese until very smooth.
- Preheat your oven to 450°F.
- Place a nonstick skillet in oven and spray with extra virgin olive oil.
- Season beef with sea salt and place in the pan; cook for about 7 minutes, turn over and cook the other side for about 4 minutes more.
- Transfer the meat to a plate and top with seasoned butter to serve.

Green Curry Beef

Total time: 1 hour, 20 minutes

Prep time: 10 minutes

Resting time: 30 minutes

Cook time: 40 minutes

Yield: 3 servings

Ingredients

- 1 tbsp. extra virgin olive oil
- ½ cup chopped parsley
- 1 cup cilantro leaves
- 1 white onion, chopped
- 1 fresh Thai green chili, chopped
- 2 cloves garlic, thinly sliced
- ¼ tsp. turmeric
- ½ tsp. ground cumin
- 2 tbsp. lime juice
- ¼ tsp. sea salt
- Black pepper
- 16 ounces beef top round, cut into small pieces
- 1 can light coconut milk
- 1/4 tsp. turmeric

- 1/2 tsp. ground cumin
- 1/4 tsp. sea salt

Directions

Green curry paste:

- In a food processor or blender, combine extra virgin olive oil, parsley, cilantro, onion, chili pepper, garlic, turmeric, cumin, lime juice, sea salt, and pepper; process until very smooth.
- Combine beef and green curry paste in a bowl; toss to coat.
- Refrigerate for at least 30 minutes.
- When ready, heat a large skillet over medium high heat and add beef along with the green curry sauce.
- Lower heat and stir for about 10 minutes or until the meat is browned on the outside.
- Stir in coconut milk and cook for about 30 minutes or until the sauce is thick.
- Serve immediately.

Roasted Pork With Balsamic Sauce

Total time: 1 hour

Prep time: 20 minutes

Cook time: 40 minutes

Yield: 6 servings

Ingredients

- 1 tsp. extra virgin olive oil
- 1 clove garlic, minced
- ¼ cup diced yellow onion
- 1 ½ cups low-sodium vegetable or chicken broth
- ¼ cup balsamic vinegar

- ½ cup port
- ¼ cup dried cherries
- ½ cup 2% milk
- ¼ cup low-fat sour cream
- ¾ lb. pork tenderloin, trimmed

Directions

- Heat extra virgin olive oil in a medium saucepan set over medium high heat; add garlic and onion and sauté for about 3 minutes or until tender.
- Stir in chicken broth, balsamic vinegar, port, and dried cherries and cook until the sauce is reduced to ½ cup.
- Scrape the sauce into the blender and blend until very smooth; stir in milk and sour cream and return to pan; stir until heated through.
- Preheat your oven to 375°F.
- Place pork tenderloin into a roasting pan and roast in the oven for about 15 minutes.
- Remove pork from oven and let rest for about 5 minutes and then slice into small slices. Serve the meat over 3 tablespoons of sauce.

Mediterranean Beef Pitas

Total time: 15 minutes

Prep time: 10 minutes

Cook time: 5 minutes

Yield: 4 servings

Ingredients

- 1 pound ground beef
- Freshly ground black pepper
- Sea salt

- 1 ½ tsp. dried oregano
- 2 tbsp. extra virgin olive oil, divided
- ¼ small red onion, sliced
- 3/4cup store-bought hummus
- 2 tbsp. fresh flat-leaf parsley
- 4 pitas
- 4 lemon wedges

Directions

- Form beef into 16 patties; season with ¼ teaspoon ground pepper, ½ teaspoon sea salt and oregano.
- Add 1 tablespoon of extra virgin olive oil in a skillet set over medium heat; cook the beef patties for about 2 minutes per side or until lightly browned.   To serve, top pitas with the beef patties, hummus, parsley and onion and drizzle with the remaining extra virgin olive oil; garnish with lemon wedges.

Parmesan Meat Loaf

Total time: 1 hour
Prep time: 10 minutes
Cook time: 50 minutes
Yield: 4 servings

Ingredients

- 1½ pounds ground beef
- ½ cup bread crumbs
- ½ cup chopped flat-leaf parsley
- 1 grated onion
- 1 large egg
- ½ cup grated Parmesan
- ¼ cup tomato paste
- Sea salt
- Freshly ground black pepper

Directions

- Preheat your oven to 400ºF. In a large bowl, mix together ground beef, bread crumbs, parsley, onion, egg, Parmesan cheese, tomato paste, sea salt and pepper.
- Line a baking sheet with foil and add the beef mixture, pressing to form an 8-inch loaf.
- Bake in the preheated oven for about 50 minutes or until cooked through.

Mediterranean Flank Steak

Total time: 1 hour
Prep time: 20 minutes
Cook time: 40 minutes
Yield: 4 to 6 servings

Ingredients

- 2 tbsp. chopped aromatic herbs (marjoram, rosemary, sage, thyme, or a mix)
- 2 cloves garlic, minced
- 2 tbsp. extra virgin olive oil
- 1 tbsp. sea salt
- 1 tbsp. ground black pepper
- 1½-to 2-lb. flank steak, trimmed
- ½ cup Greek vinaigrette

Directions

- In a small bowl, mix together herbs, garlic, extra virgin olive oil, sea salt, and pepper; rub over the steak and let rest for about 20 minutes.
- In the meantime, heat your gas grill to medium high.

- Grill the steak for about 15 minutes, turning meat every 4 minutes for even cooking.
- Transfer the cooked steak to a cutting board and let rest for about 5 minutes; slice into small slices and place on plates.
- Drizzle with vinaigrette and serve immediately.

Mediterranean Lamb Chops

Total time: 1 hour 30

Prep time: 30 minutes

Cook time: 1 hour

Yield: 4 servings

Ingredients

- 2 tbsp. extra virgin olive oil, divided
- 3 garlic cloves
- 1 tsp. chopped fresh rosemary
- 2 tbsp. chopped fresh mint
- 4 lean lamb chops
- 2 yellow peppers, diced
- 2 red peppers, diced
- 4 zucchinis, sliced
- 1 eggplant, sliced
- 3 oz. crumbled feta cheese
- 9 oz. cherry tomatoes

Directions

- Preheat your oven to 350ºF.
- In a food processor, blend together 1 tablespoon extra virgin olive oil, garlic, rosemary, and mint until very smooth; smear over the lamb chops.
- On a baking sheet, mix peppers, zucchini, and eggplant; drizzle with the remaining oil.
- Place the lamb chops over the vegetables and roast in the preheated oven for about 25 minutes.
- Remove the baking sheet from oven and top with cherry tomatoes and feta cheese; return to oven and continue roasting for 10 minutes more or until lamb chops are cooked through and cheese begins to brown.
- Serve the roasted vegetables with lamb chops and green salad.

LAMB EXOHIKO

Serves 4

- 2 tablespoons extra-virgin olive oil
- 4 cups fresh spinach, blanched, drained, and chopped 4 or 5 scallions, ends trimmed and chopped
- 1 clove garlic, peeled and minced
- 1/4 cup dry white wine
- 3/4 teaspoon salt 1/2 teaspoon pepper
- 2 tablespoons chopped fresh dill
- 1 teaspoon dried oregano
- 8 sheets phyllo pastry, thawed, at room temperature
- 1/2 cup melted butter 2 cups diced cooked lamb meat
- 4 (1/4-inch) slices ripe medium-size tomato
- 4 (1/4-inch) slices kefalotyri or Romano cheese

- 4 (¼-inch) slices red bell pepper, stemmed and seeded

Directions

- Heat the oil in a large skillet over medium heat for 30 seconds. Add the spinach, scallions, and garlic, and cook for 5–6 minutes. Add the wine, and cook for 2–3 minutes to reduce the wine. Season with salt and pepper. Add the dill and oregano, take the skillet off the heat, and reserve.
- Preheat the oven to 350°F. Place the phyllo on a clean work surface, and cover sheets with a lightly damp tea towel to keep them from drying. Brush a sheet of phyllo with butter. Take a second sheet, place it on top of the first sheet, and brush it with butter.
- Place one-fourth of the lamb on the phyllo about 5 inches from the bottom and leave 2 inches from the left and the right sides. Top the lamb with one-fourth of the spinach filling, a slice of tomato, a slice of cheese, and a slice of red pepper. Fold the bottom 5 inches of phyllo over the filling, and then fold in the left and right sides. Next, roll the phyllo to make a bundle. Place the bundle, seam-side down, on a baking sheet lined with parchment paper. Repeat this process three more times.
- Brush the tops of the bundles with butter, and bake them on the middle rack for 25–30 minutes or until they are golden.
- Serve immediately or warm.

LEMON VERBENA RACK OF LAMB

Serves 4

- 2 (2-pound) racks lamb, silver skin removed and tied
- ¼ cup extra-virgin olive oil
- 2 cloves garlic, peeled and crushed
- 1 tablespoon Dijon mustard
- 1 teaspoon sweet paprika
- 1 tablespoon honey
- 2 teaspoons grated lemon zest
- 2 tablespoons chopped fresh parsley
- 2 tablespoons lemon verbena leaves
- 2 teaspoons fresh thyme leaves
- 3 teaspoons salt
- 1 teaspoon pepper

Directions

- Place the lamb in a medium baking dish. In a food processor, put the oil, garlic, mustard, paprika, honey, zest, parsley, lemon verbena, and thyme. Process until the ingredients are well incorporated. Pour the marinade over the lamb and rub it all over to coat. Cover and marinate the lamb for 1 hour at room temperature. Season the lamb with salt and pepper.
- Preheat the broiler. Place the lamb on a baking tray lined with parchment paper and roast it under the broiler for 5 minutes. Set the oven temperature to 450°F and roast for 25 minutes. Check the internal temperature of the lamb; it should read a minimum of 135°F. If you

prefer the meat well done, roast the lamb for a few more minutes.

- Tent the lamb with foil and let it rest for 5 minutes before serving.

- Ask the butcher to trim the rack of lamb and remove its silver skin. He or she will then tie the lamb into a crown rack, which will save some preparation time.

TANGY MAPLE-MUSTARD LAMB

Serves 6

- 3 pounds lamb chops
- 1⁄4 cup extra-virgin olive oil 2 tablespoons chopped fresh rosemary
- 2 cloves garlic, peeled and minced
- 1 teaspoon pepper
- 1 tablespoon Dijon mustard
- 1⁄4 cup maple syrup 1 teaspoon orange zest
- 2 teaspoons salt
- 3 tablespoons vegetable oil
- 1 large lemon, cut into wedges

Directions

- Put the lamb in a medium baking dish. In a medium bowl, whisk the oil, rosemary, garlic, pepper, mustard, maple syrup, and orange zest. Reserve 1⁄3 cup of the marinade to brush on the lamb after grilling. Pour the remaining marinade over the lamb and rub it all over to coat. Cover and marinate for 1 hour at room temperature or refrigerate overnight. Bring the lamb to room temperature, if it

was refrigerated. Season the lamb with salt.

- Preheat the gas or charcoal grill to medium-high. Brush the grill surface to make sure it is thoroughly clean. When the grill is ready, dip a clean tea towel in the vegetable oil and wipe the grill's surface with the oil.

- Place the lamb on the grill, and grill it 3–4 minutes a side for medium- rare or 4 minutes a side for medium. Brush the reserved marinade on the lamb chops and let them rest for 5 minutes.

- Serve the lamb with the lemon wedges.

OSSO BUCO

Serves 10

- 5 pounds veal shanks
- 2 teaspoons salt, divided
- 1 teaspoon pepper, divided
- 1 tablespoon extra-virgin olive oil
- 1 leek, ends trimmed, thoroughly cleaned, cut lengthwise, and sliced
- 3 large tomatoes, cut into wedges
- 4 medium onions, peeled and cut into large wedges
- 4 cloves garlic, peeled and smashed
- 2 stalks celery, ends trimmed and cut into chunks
- 2 medium carrots, peeled and cut into chunks
- 1 cup dry red wine
- 3 cups veal or beef stock
- 2 bay leaves
- 3 tablespoons chopped fresh parsley

- 1 tablespoon fresh thyme leaves
- 1 tablespoon chopped fresh rosemary

Directions

- Preheat the oven to 325°F. Season the shanks with 1 teaspoon of salt and 1/2 teaspoon of pepper.
- Heat the oil in a Dutch oven (with a lid) over medium-high heat for 30 seconds. Add the shanks and brown them for 3–4 minutes on both sides.
- Add the leeks, tomatoes, onions, garlic, celery, and carrots. Brown the vegetables lightly. Add the wine and cook it for 2–3 minutes to let it reduce by half.
- Add the stock, bay leaves, parsley, thyme, and rosemary. Bring the veal to a boil, cover it immediately, and place it in the oven. Braise the dish for 2–3 hours, until the meat is fork-tender and starts to separate from the bone. Remove the bay leaves.
- Serve it hot or let it come to room temperature, refrigerate it, and reheat it the next day.

HÜNKAR BEGENDI WITH LAMB

Serves 6

- 2 pounds cubed lamb meat, rinsed and dried
- 2 1/2 teaspoons salt, divided
- 1 teaspoon pepper, divided
- 2 tablespoons olive oil
- 1 large onion, peeled and thinly sliced

- 1/2 cup diced green pepper, stemmed and seeded 3 or 4 cloves garlic, peeled and minced
- 2 or 3 bay leaves
- 6 or 7 whole allspice berries
- 2 tablespoons puréed roasted red peppers
- 2 teaspoons fresh thyme leaves
- 2 tablespoons chopped fresh parsley
- 2 cups puréed tomatoes
- 2 cups hot water or lamb stock
- 2 large eggplants, charred and flesh reserved
- 2 tablespoons unsalted butter
- 2 tablespoons all-purpose flour
- 2 cups whole milk
- 1/2 cup grated kefalotyri or Romano cheese
- 3 tablespoons cream cheese
- 1/2 cup chopped fresh chives

Directions

- Season the lamb with 1 teaspoon of salt and 1/2 teaspoon pepper. Heat the oil in a large skillet over medium-high heat for 30 seconds. Add the lamb cubes and brown them for 2–3 minutes on all sides. Add the onions, green peppers, garlic, bay leaves, and allspice, and reduce the heat to medium. Cook for 6–7 minutes.
- Add the red peppers, thyme, parsley, tomatoes, and hot water or stock. Increase the heat to medium-high, and bring the mixture to a boil. Reduce the heat to medium, partially cover the skillet, and cook for 30– 40 minutes.

Uncover, season with 1 teaspoon of salt and 1⁄4 teaspoon of pepper, and continue to cook until the sauce thickens. Take the skillet off the heat and keep warm.

- Put the eggplant flesh in a mortar, and pound it with the pestle until it becomes creamy but still chunky. Reserve.
- Melt the butter in a medium saucepan over medium heat. Add the flour and stir the mixture until it turns light brown. Continue to stir and slowly add the milk. Keep stirring until the milk thickens. Stir in the reserved eggplant and cheeses. Season with the remaining salt and pepper.
- Serve a generous ladle of eggplant sauce on each plate and top with the lamb. Sprinkle the chives on top and serve warm.

MOUSSAKA

Serves 10

- 2 tablespoons salt
- 3 large eggplants, ends trimmed and cut into 1⁄2-inch slices
- 1⁄2 cup extra-virgin olive oil
- 1 cup bread crumbs, divided
- 6 cups Greek Meat Sauce
- 11⁄2 cups grated kefalotyri or Romano cheese, divided 4 cups Béchamel Sauce

Directions

- Sprinkle the salt over the eggplant slices, and leave them for 30 minutes to release their bitter liquid. Wipe the eggplants dry with a paper towel. Preheat the oven to 400°F.

- Brush the eggplants with oil and place them on a baking sheet. Bake the eggplants for 6 minutes until softened. (The eggplant can also be grilled.) Transfer the eggplant to a tray lined with paper towels to soak up excess oil, and let them cool. Reduce the oven temperature to 375°F.

- In a large casserole dish, place a layer of the eggplant on the bottom. Sprinkle 1⁄2 cup of bread crumbs over the eggplant. Spread half of the Greek Meat Sauce over the bread crumbs. Next sprinkle 1⁄2 cup cheese over the top. Add another layer of eggplant, the remaining bread crumbs, Greek Meat Sauce, and 1⁄2 cup of cheese.

- Top the moussaka with the Béchamel Sauce. Sprinkle the remaining cheese on top, and bake for 30–40 minutes or until the top is golden.

- Allow the moussaka to rest for 45 minutes before cutting and serving.

SLOW-COOKED PORK CHOPS IN WINE

Serves 4

- 1⁄4 cup all-purpose flour
- 11⁄2 teaspoons salt
- 1⁄2 teaspoon pepper
- 2 teaspoons sweet paprika
- 4 bone-in pork chops, rinsed and dried
- 1⁄4 cup extra-virgin olive oil

- 1/2 cup dry white wine
- 1 cup Chicken or Turkey Stock or Basic Vegetable Stock
- 2 bay leaves
- 6–8 large green olives, pitted and chopped
- 1 tablespoon fresh lemon juice
- 1 tablespoon fresh thyme leaves

Directions

- Combine the flour, salt, pepper, and paprika in a medium bowl. Stir to combine the ingredients. Dredge the pork chops in the flour. Reserve the pork chops and discard the flour.
- Heat the oil in a large skillet over medium-high heat for 30 seconds. Add the pork chops and brown them for 2–3 minutes per side. Remove the pork chops and reserve.
- Add the wine, stock, and bay leaves. Stir and cook the sauce for 2–3 minutes, scraping up brown bits from the bottom of the pan. Put the pork chops back in the skillet. Cover it, and reduce the heat to medium-low. Cook for 30 minutes or until the pork is tender and the sauce has reduced by half.
- Add the olives, lemon juice, and thyme. Season with more salt and pepper, if necessary.
- Remove the bay leaves and serve.

PORK CHOPS IN WINE

Serves 4

4 thick-cut pork chops

- 1/2 cup extra-virgin olive oil
- 1 cup white wine
- 1/2 cup hot water
- 1 tablespoon dried oregano Salt and pepper to taste

Directions

- Rinse pork chops well and pat dry with a paper towel.
- Place 2 tablespoons olive oil in a frying pan; lightly brown pork chops.
- Put remaining olive oil in a fresh pan and turn heat to medium-high. Cook pork chops 3–4 minutes per side, making sure to turn them over at least once.
- Add wine; bring to a boil. Turn to medium and simmer for 10 minutes, turning the meat once.
- Add 1/2 cup hot water to pan; bring to a boil and let simmer until the sauce has reduced. Sprinkle with oregano, salt, and pepper, and serve immediately.

BREADED PORK CHOPS

Serves 6

- 3 slices raisin-pumpernickel bread
- 6 cloves garlic
- 1/2 cup applesauce 1 teaspoon olive oil
- 6 pork chops
- Fresh-cracked black pepper, to taste
- Kosher salt, to taste

Directions

- Preheat oven to 375°F. Spray a baking sheet with cooking spray.
- Toast the bread and grate into crumbs. Mince the garlic in a blender, then add

the applesauce and oil, and blend until smooth.

- Rub the chops with the garlic-applesauce mixture. Bread with pumpernickel crumbs and place on prepared baking sheet. Spray the chops with cooking spray and season with pepper and salt.

- Bake for 20 minutes, then turn and bake for 20–40 minutes longer, depending on the thickness of the pork. Serve hot.

SMYRNA SOUTZOUKAKIA

Serves 4

- 2 slices white bread
- 1/2 cup white wine, divided
- 1 pound lean ground beef
- 2 medium onions, peeled (1 grated, 1 diced), divided 4 cloves garlic, minced, divided
- 3 tablespoons finely chopped fresh parsley
- 1/2 teaspoon plus 1/8 teaspoon ground cumin, divided 1 teaspoon dried oregano
- 2 1/2 teaspoons salt, divided 3/4 teaspoon pepper, divided 1 large egg, beaten
- 1/2 cup extra-virgin olive oil, divided
- 1 bay leaf
- 1 (28-ounce) can plum tomatoes, puréed
- 1/8 teaspoon cinnamon

Directions

- Soak the bread in 1/4 cup of the wine, squeeze out the liquid, and crumble the bread. In a large bowl, mix the beef, bread, grated onion, 1 teaspoon of the garlic, parsley, 1/2 teaspoon of the

cumin, oregano, 2 teaspoons of the salt, 1/2 teaspoon of the pepper, and the egg. Mix well and refrigerate for 1 hour.

- Heat 1/4 cup of the oil in a medium skillet over medium-high heat for 30 seconds. Add the diced onions, bay leaf, tomatoes, remaining garlic, remaining cumin, cinnamon, and remaining wine. Season with the remaining salt and pepper. Reduce the heat to medium-low and cook for 30 minutes.

- Form the meat mixture into 3-inch, quenelle-shaped sausages. Preheat a gas or charcoal grill to medium-high. Place the sausages on the grill and grill them 3–4 minutes a side (if you prefer to fry them instead, lightly dredge them in flour before frying them in olive oil).

- Place the sausages in the tomato sauce and cook for 10–15 minutes.

- Remove the bay leaf and serve hot.

STUFFED PEPPERS WITH MEAT

Serves 6

- 1/3 cup extra-virgin olive oil 2 medium onions, peeled and diced
- 3 cloves garlic, peeled and minced
- 1 cup finely chopped fresh parsley
- 1 cup finely chopped fresh dill
- 2 tablespoons finely chopped fresh mint
- 1 cup tomato sauce
- 1 cup long-grain rice
- 2 pounds lean ground beef
- 2 1/2 teaspoons salt

- ¾ teaspoon pepper 2–3 cups hot water

Directions

- Preheat the oven to 375°F. Heat the oil in a large skillet over medium-high heat for 30 seconds. Reduce the heat to medium, and add the onions and garlic. Cook for 10 minutes or until the onions soften. Add the parsley, dill, mint, and tomato sauce. Cook for 10 minutes or until the sauce thickens. Take the skillet off the heat and cool it for 5 minutes.
- Add the rice and ground beef to the skillet. Season with the salt and pepper and cook until rice is soft and beef is browned.
- Spoon the beef-rice mixture into the peppers and place them in a roasting pan that will hold all the peppers snugly. Add 2–3 cups of hot water, enough to fill the pan up to 1 inch on the sides of the peppers.
- Bake on the middle rack of the oven for 70–80 minutes or until the pepper tops are golden and the rice is cooked.
- Serve hot or at room temperature.

ROAST PORK BELLY AND POTATOES

Serves 12

- 10–12 medium Yukon gold potatoes, peeled and quartered
- ½ cup extra-virgin olive oil
- ½ cup hot Chicken or Turkey Stock or Basic Vegetable Stock
- 2 tablespoons Dijon mustard
- 1 tablespoon lemon juice
- 10 sprigs fresh thyme plus
- 2 teaspoons fresh thyme leaves, divided
- 2 or 3 sprigs fresh rosemary
- 3 teaspoons salt, divided
- 1½ teaspoons pepper, divided
- 1 (3½-pound) pork belly, cut into ½-inch slices
- 2 teaspoons sweet paprika
- 1 teaspoon dried oregano
- ¼ cup diced smoked pork or bacon
- 1 head garlic, top third cut off

Directions

- Preheat the oven to 400°F. In a roasting pan, put the potatoes, olive oil, stock, mustard, lemon juice, thyme sprigs, and rosemary. Toss to combine the ingredients and coat the potatoes. Season with 1 teaspoon of salt and ½ teaspoon of pepper and toss again. Reserve.
- In a large bowl, combine the pork belly, remaining salt, remaining pepper, paprika, oregano, and thyme leaves. Toss to combine the ingredients and coat the pork.
- Place the pork belly on the potatoes. Sprinkle the smoked pork over the potatoes and the pork belly. Nestle the garlic in the middle of the pan.
- Bake on the middle rack for 30 minutes or until the tops of the pork are nicely browned. Turn the pork belly over and bake for another 20 minutes or until the

pork is browned and the potatoes are cooked.

- Serve immediately.

GREEK-STYLE RIBS

Serves 4

- 1 tablespoon onion powder
- 1 tablespoon garlic powder
- 2 tablespoons lemon pepper
- 1 teaspoon ground bay
- 1 teaspoon dry oregano
- 1 teaspoon dry thyme
- 1 tablespoon seasoning salt
- 2 tablespoons sweet paprika
- 2 racks pork baby-back ribs, silver skin removed

Directions

- In a medium bowl, combine all the ingredients except the ribs. Rub the mix evenly over the ribs. Refrigerate for 3 hours or let sit for 1 hour at room temperature. Preheat the oven to 425°F.
- Bring ribs to room temperature. Place them on a baking sheet lined with parchment paper. Cover with foil and bake for 45 minutes; lower the heat to 375°F and bake for 15 minutes. Remove foil and bake for another 30 minutes. Tent the ribs with foil for 5 minutes. Cut ribs and serve.

GRILLED LAMB CHOPS

Serves 4

- 1⁄2 cup extra-virgin olive oil
- 3 cloves garlic, peeled and minced
- 1 teaspoon Dijon mustard
- 2 tablespoons chopped fresh parsley
- 1 tablespoon fresh thyme leaves
- 1 tablespoon fresh lemon juice
- 2 teaspoons pepper
- 2 1⁄2 teaspoons salt
- 2 teaspoons dried oregano, divided
- 2 1⁄2 pounds lamb chops
- 3 tablespoons vegetable oil
- 1 large lemon, cut into wedges

Directions

- In a small bowl, thoroughly whisk the olive oil, garlic, mustard, parsley, thyme, lemon juice, pepper, salt, and 1 teaspoon of oregano. Reserve one-third of the marinade to brush on the lamb after grilling.
- Place the lamb in a medium baking dish and top with two-thirds of the marinade. Rub the lamb to coat it in the marinade. Cover and refrigerate for 2 hours. Return the lamb to room temperature before grilling.
- Preheat a gas or charcoal grill to medium-high heat. Brush the grill surface to make sure it is clean. When the grill is ready, dip a clean tea towel in the vegetable oil and wipe the grill surface with the oil. Place the lamb on the grill and cook for 3–4 minutes a side for medium-rare and 4 minutes a side for medium. Brush the reserved marinade on the lamb and let the chops rest for 5 minutes.

- Sprinkle the chops with the remaining oregano and serve with the lemon wedges.

KONTOSOUVLI

Serves 10
- 1 medium onion, peeled and grated
- 2 or 3 cloves garlic, peeled and minced
- 1 tablespoon sweet paprika
- 2 teaspoons fresh thyme leaves
- 3 tablespoons dried oregano
- 1/2 cup dry red wine 1 1/2 teaspoons pepper
- 3 teaspoons salt, divided
- 6 pound pork butt, cut into 4-inch chunks
- 2 large lemons, cut into wedges

Directions

- In a large bowl, whisk the onions, garlic, paprika, thyme, oregano, red wine, pepper, and 2 teaspoons of salt. Add the pork; toss to combine the ingredients and coat the pork. Cover and refrigerate overnight. Bring the pork to room temperature before grilling.
- Prepare the rotisserie. If using a charcoal pit, bring it to a medium heat. If using a gas grill, remove the grates and place a drip pan with water beneath the rotisserie. The drip pan will keep the grill clean and prevent flare-ups as the fat renders.
- Skewer the meat (close to each other) on the rotisserie spit and secure at each end. Season the meat with the remaining salt. Put the spit over the heat and grill.

Lower the lid on a gas grill. Check and replenish the drip pan with water every 1/2 hour (the charcoal grill doesn't need a drip pan).
- After 1 hour, begin slicing off some of the outer layers of meat. Continue slicing off meat as the Kontosouvli cooks. Serve it with the lemon wedges.

PORK SOUVLAKI

Serves 8
- 1 large onion, peeled and grated
- 3 cloves garlic, peeled and minced
- 2 teaspoons salt
- 3/4 teaspoon pepper
- 1/4 cup plus 3 tablespoons vegetable oil, divided
- 4 teaspoons dried oregano, divided
- 2 pound boneless pork butt, fat trimmed and cut into 1-inch cubes 2 large lemons, cut into wedges

Directions

- In a large bowl, whisk the onion, garlic, salt, pepper, 1/4 cup oil, and oregano. Whisk to thoroughly combine the marinade. Add the pork and toss to coat the meat. Refrigerate the pork for at least 5 hours or overnight. Bring the pork to room temperature before grilling it.
- Put the meat onto wooden or metal skewers. Add 4 pieces of pork per skewer.
- Preheat the gas or charcoal grill to medium-high. Brush the grill surface to make sure it is thoroughly clean. When

the grill is ready, dip a clean tea towel in the remaining oil and wipe the grill surface with the oil. Put the pork on the grill and cook it for 3–4 minutes a side or until the pork is cooked through.

- Sprinkle the pork with the remaining oregano and serve it with the lemon wedges.

SPETSOFAI

Serves 4

- 1/4 cup extra-virgin olive oil, divided 4 (5-inch) fresh sausages
- 4 hot banana peppers, stemmed, seeded, and skins pierced 2 large red or yellow bell peppers, stemmed, seeded, and sliced 2 medium onions, peeled and sliced
- 3 or 4 cloves garlic, peeled and minced
- 2 large ripe tomatoes, skinned and grated
- 1/2 teaspoon salt
- 1/2 teaspoon pepper
- 2 teaspoons dry oregano

Directions

- Heat 2 tablespoons of oil in a large skillet over medium-high heat for 30 seconds. Add the sausages and brown them for 2–3 minutes on all sides. Remove the sausages from the skillet and reserve.
- Add the banana peppers and fry them on all sides until they are just brown, about 60–90 seconds per side. Remove the banana peppers and reserve.

- Add the bell peppers, onions, garlic, and tomatoes. Bring the mixture to a boil and then reduce the heat to medium-low. Season it with salt and pepper. Return the sausages and banana peppers to the skillet. Cover and cook for 15–20 minutes or until the sauce thickens.
- Remove the cover and add the oregano. Adjust the seasoning with salt and pepper, if necessary. Drizzle the remaining oil over the dish. Serve hot.

FASOLAKIA WITH VEAL

Serves 4

- 1/3 cup extra-virgin olive oil 3 medium onions, peeled and sliced
- 5 cloves garlic, peeled and sliced
- 1/2 cup chopped fresh parsley
- 1/4 cup finely chopped fresh mint
- 1/2 cup chopped fresh dill 2 pounds fasolakia (runner beans), trimmed
- 3 large ripe tomatoes, skinned and grated
- 1 teaspoon salt
- 1/2 teaspoon pepper 2 pounds cooked veal or beef, cut into bite-size pieces
- 2 large potatoes, peeled and quartered
- 2–3 cups hot veal broth

Directions

- Heat the oil in a large skillet over medium-high heat for 30 seconds. Add the onions and cook for 5 minutes or until they soften. Add the garlic, parsley, mint, dill, beans, and tomatoes. Bring the mixture to a boil and then reduce the heat to medium-low and cook for 30 minutes. Season with salt and pepper.

- Add the veal, potatoes, and enough broth just to cover the ingredients. Cook for another 30 minutes or until the potatoes are cooked and the sauce thickens a little.

- Adjust the seasoning with more salt and pepper, if necessary. Serve hot.

SLOW-ROASTED LEG OF LAMB

Serves 10

- 1 (6–8 pound) leg of lamb, bone in
- 1 head garlic, cloves peeled and sliced thinly
- 3 tablespoons extra-virgin olive oil
- 5 teaspoons salt
- 2 teaspoons pepper
- 2 teaspoons garlic powder
- 2 teaspoons sweet paprika
- 2 medium onions, peeled and quartered
- 2 or 3 sprigs fresh rosemary
- 10 sprigs fresh thyme
- 2–3 teaspoons dried oregano
- 2 or 3 bay leaves
- 1/3 cup fresh lemon juice
- 1 cup dry white wine Hot water

Directions

- Stick a paring knife into the lamb and make a hole; then slip a sliver of garlic into the hole. Repeat this process and insert as many slivers of garlic as you can into the leg.

- Preheat the oven to 550°F or its highest temperature. Put the lamb in a roasting

pan (that just fits the lamb) and rub 3 tablespoons of oil all over it. Season all sides with the salt, pepper, garlic powder, and paprika.

- Roast the lamb uncovered for 10–15 minutes or until browned. Flip the lamb over and roast it on the other side for 10–15 minutes or until browned. Remove the pan from the oven. Reduce the oven temperature to 350°F.

- To the roasting pan, add the onions, any remaining slivers of garlic, rosemary, thyme, oregano, and bay leaves. Add the lemon juice, wine, and just enough hot water to rise one-third of the way up the lamb. Cover and roast the lamb for 2 hours. Baste the lamb after the first hour.

- Turn the lamb over and roast for another hour. Add more hot water if necessary. The lamb should be deep brown, the bone will be exposed, and the meat should be separating from the bone.

- Remove the bay leaves. Baste the lamb, and let it rest for 15–20 minutes before serving.

BRAISED SHORT RIBS KOKKINISTO

Serves 4

- 4 (8-ounce) thick beef short ribs
- 1 1/2 teaspoons salt 1/2 teaspoon pepper 1/4 cup all-purpose flour 1/2 cup extra-virgin olive oil, divided 1/2 stalk celery, ends trimmed and diced 1/2 medium carrot, peeled and diced 3 medium

onions, peeled (1 whole, 1 diced), divided 5 or 6 cloves garlic, peeled

- 6 whole allspice berries
- 2 bay leaves
- 1 teaspoon smoked paprika
- 1⁄2 cup dry white wine 2 tablespoons tomato paste
- 1 teaspoon fresh thyme leaves
- 1 teaspoon fresh rosemary leaves
- 2 cups hot water

Directions

- Season beef with salt and pepper and dredge in flour. In an ovenproof pot, just big enough to hold the ribs, heat 2 tablespoons of oil over medium-high heat for 30 seconds. Add the beef (in batches) and brown for 3 minutes on each side. Remove the beef and reserve.
- Add the remaining oil to the pan and reduce heat to medium. Add celery, carrots, onions, garlic, allspice, bay leaves, and paprika. Stir and cook for 5–6 minutes to soften the vegetables. Preheat the oven to 350°F.
- Add the wine and allow it to reduce for 3 minutes. Add the tomato paste, thyme, and rosemary. Return the beef to the pan and add the hot water. Cover and bake for 70–90 minutes.
- Check the seasoning and adjust with salt and pepper, if necessary. Return the pot to the oven and bake for 30 minutes. Remove from the oven and uncover; remove the bay leaves. Serve hot.

LAMB ON THE SPIT

Serves 30

- 1 (15–20 pound) whole lamb
- 1⁄2 cup vegetable oil 1 1⁄2 cups salt, divided 6 tablespoons pepper, divided
- 1⁄2 cup garlic powder
- 1⁄4 cup lemon juice
- 3⁄4 cup extra-virgin olive oil
- 1⁄2 cup dried oregano
- 1⁄2 cup Ladolemono

Directions

- Place the spit rod through the lamb (rear to head). If the head is still on the lamb, pierce the skull to help secure the spit. Break the hind legs, bending them backward, and tie them securely to the spit with butcher's twine. Repeat this step with the front legs and also securely bind the neck to the spit. Using butcher's twine and an upholstery needle, make a stitch across the length of the lamb's spine, looping around the spit. It's important that the stitch enters the meat near the spine, loops around the spit, and then the needle comes back out of the body near the spine again. Loop the twine through your stitch and continue securing the spine to the spit until you've reached the shoulder.
- Rub the inside of the lamb with vegetable oil and sprinkle with 1⁄2 cup salt, 3 tablespoons pepper, and garlic powder. Using the butcher's twine and needle, stitch and close the opening to the cavity. Rub the exterior of the lamb with oil and

season it well with 3⁄4 cup salt and remaining pepper.

- Get a fire pit started with some kindling wood and newspaper. When some burning embers are present, add two bags of charcoal into the pit and allow 30 minutes for the charcoal to get white-hot.

- Separate the hot coals into two piles: one underneath the shoulder end, and the other pile under the hind leg side. The midsection of the lamb cooks the fastest and there is enough residual heat from both piles to cook the midsection evenly. Every hour, replenish the pit with another bag of charcoal, with two piles at each end of the pit. When the older charcoals start losing heat, just push the newer charcoals over to the two main charcoal areas. The lamb should take 5–6 hours to cook through.

- In a medium bowl, combine the lemon juice, olive oil, remaining salt, and oregano to make a basting marinade. Baste frequently for the last hour. The lamb will show signs of being done when the carcass starts to crack.

- Transfer the lamb to a large baking tray, allow it to rest 15–20 minutes, and then cut away all butcher's twine and carve it into pieces. Drizzle the Ladolemono on the meat before serving.

CABBAGE ROLLS

Serves 10

- 1⁄4 cup extra-virgin olive oil 3 medium onions, finely diced
- 3 cloves garlic, minced
- 1⁄4 cup tomato purée 1 pound lean ground beef
- 1 pound ground pork
- 11⁄2 cups Arborio rice 1 cup chopped fresh parsley
- 1 cup chopped fresh dill
- 3 teaspoons salt
- 1 teaspoon black pepper
- 1 large cabbage, blanched, leaves separated and trimmed
- 3 cups Chicken or Turkey Stock or Basic Vegetable Stock
- 4 tablespoons all-purpose flour
- 2 tablespoons water
- 3 large eggs
- 6 tablespoons fresh lemon juice

Directions

- Heat the oil in a large skillet over medium-high heat. Reduce the heat to medium and add the onions and garlic. Cook for 10 minutes or until the onions soften. Take the skillet off the heat and stir in the tomato purée, beef, pork, rice, parsley, dill, salt, and pepper.

- Place a cabbage leaf on a work surface. Add a generous tablespoon of filling near the bottom of the leaf. Fold the two ends of the leaf inward and roll it into a long, narrow bundle. Do not roll the leaf too tightly or the rice will break the cabbage as it expands. Repeat the process until all the filling is used.

- Preheat the oven to 350°F. Place some leftover leaves on the bottom of a roasting pan. Place the cabbage rolls in concentric circles in the pan. Top with more loose cabbage leaves. Add the stock, cover, and bake on the lower rack for 90 minutes. Carefully pour any remaining liquid from the pan into a bowl. Reserve.

- In a large bowl, whisk the flour and water to form a slurry. Whisk in the eggs and lemon juice. Continuing to whisk vigorously, slowly add a ladle of cabbage-roll liquid into the egg-lemon mixture. Continue whisking and slowly add another two ladles (one at a time) into the egg-lemon mixture.

- Pour the avgolemono over the rolls and shake the pan to allow the sauce to blend in. Let the dish cool for 15 minutes before serving.

ZUCCHINI STUFFED WITH MEAT AND RICE

Serves 6

- 1⁄4 cup extra-virgin olive oil 2 medium onions, peeled and finely diced
- 3 cloves garlic, peeled and minced
- 1 1⁄2 cups chopped fresh parsley 3⁄4 cup chopped fresh dill 1⁄2 cup chopped fresh mint 2⁄3 cup tomato sauce
- 1⁄4 cup plus 2 tablespoons water plus 3 cups hot water, divided
- 1 1⁄2 cups Arborio rice 2 pounds extra-lean ground beef
- 1 tablespoon salt

- 3⁄4 teaspoon black pepper 10 medium zucchini, peeled, cut in half, and cored
- 4 tablespoons all-purpose flour
- 3 large eggs
- 6 tablespoons fresh lemon juice

Directions

- Preheat the oven to 375°F. Heat the oil in a large skillet over medium-high heat for 30 seconds. Reduce the heat to medium and add the onions and garlic. Cook for 5–6 minutes or until the onions soften. Stir in the parsley, dill, and mint. Add the tomato sauce, 1⁄4 cup of water, and the rice. Cook for 10 minutes while stirring. Stir in the beef, salt, and pepper. Take the skillet off the heat.

- Stuff the zucchini with the filling. Place them in a roasting pan big enough to hold them in a single layer. Pour 3 cups of hot water into the roasting pan, cover it with a lid, and bake for 60 minutes. Carefully tilt the roasting pan and pour any remaining liquid from the pan into a bowl.

- Reserve the liquid and the zucchini.

- In a large bowl, whisk the flour and 2 tablespoons of water to form a slurry. Whisk in the eggs and lemon juice. Continuing to whisk vigorously, slowly add a ladle of the reserved liquid into the egg-lemon mixture. Continue whisking and slowly add another 2 ladles (one at a time) into the egg-lemon mixture. Adjust the seasoning with salt, if necessary.

- Pour the avgolemono over the zucchini and shake the pan to allow the sauce to blend in. Let it cool for 15 minutes before serving warm.

GREEK-STYLE FLANK STEAK

Serves 4

- 1⁄4 cup extra-virgin olive oil 7 or 8 cloves garlic, peeled and smashed
- 4 or 5 chopped scallions, ends trimmed
- 1 tablespoon Dijon mustard
- 1⁄3 cup balsamic vinegar 2 bay leaves
- 2 tablespoons fresh thyme leaves
- 2 tablespoons fresh rosemary leaves
- 1 teaspoon dried oregano
- 1 1⁄2 teaspoons salt, divided 3⁄4 teaspoon pepper, divided 1 (2-pound) large flank steak
- 3 tablespoons vegetable oil

Directions

- In a food processor, process the olive oil, garlic, scallions, mustard, vinegar, bay leaves, thyme, rosemary, oregano, 1 teaspoon salt, and 1⁄2 teaspoon pepper. Thoroughly incorporate the ingredients in the marinade.
- Rub the steak with the marinade and place in a medium baking dish. Cover and refrigerate for 3 hours. Return the steak to room temperature before grilling. Wipe most of the marinade off the steak and season with remaining salt and pepper.
- Preheat a gas or charcoal grill to medium-high. Brush the grill surface to make sure it is thoroughly clean. When the grill is ready, dip a clean tea towel in the vegetable oil and wipe the grill surface with the oil. Place the meat on the grill and grill for 4 minutes a side.
- Let the steak rest for 5 minutes before serving.

CHEESE-STUFFED BIFTEKI

Serves 6

- 2 pounds medium ground beef
- 2 medium onions, peeled and grated
- 3 slices of bread, soaked in water, hand squeezed, and crumbled
- 1 tablespoon minced garlic
- 1 teaspoon dried oregano
- 1 teaspoon chopped fresh parsley
- 1⁄4 teaspoon ground allspice 2 tablespoons salt
- 1 teaspoon pepper
- 6 (1-inch) cubes Graviera cheese
- 3 tablespoons vegetable oil

Directions

- In a large bowl, combine all the ingredients (except the cheese and vegetable oil) and mix thoroughly.
- Using your hands, form twelve (4" × 1⁄2") patties with the meat. Place the patties on a tray, cover them with plastic wrap, and refrigerate for 4 hours or overnight. Allow the patties to come to room temperature before grilling.
- Take a piece of cheese and place it on the middle of a patty. Place another patty on top and press them together to form one burger. Using your fingers, pinch the entire perimeter of the burger so that

when you grill, the burger will hold together and the cheese will not leak out.

- Preheat a gas or charcoal grill to medium-high. Brush the grill surface to make sure it is thoroughly clean. When the grill is ready, dip a clean tea towel in the vegetable oil and wipe the grill surface with the oil. Place the burgers on the grill and grill for 5 minutes a side.
- Allow the burgers to rest for 5 minutes before serving.

MEATBALLS IN EGG-LEMON SAUCE

Serves 6

- 2 pounds lean ground veal
- 2 medium onions, finely diced
- 1/2 cup dry bread crumbs 1 egg, beaten, plus 2 eggs
- 1/4 cup extra-virgin olive oil, divided
- 1/4 cup fresh mint, finely chopped
- 1/4 cup fresh parsley, finely chopped
- 1 teaspoon dried oregano
- Salt and pepper to taste
- 4 cups Beef Stock or Veal Stock Juice of 1 lemon

Directions

- Preheat the oven to 400°F.
- In a large mixing bowl, combine meat, onions, bread crumbs, 1 beaten egg, 2 tablespoons olive oil, mint, parsley, oregano, salt, and pepper; mix together well with your hands.
- Using your fingers, take up small pieces of meat mix and fashion into meatballs

about the size of a golf ball. Place in rows in a baking dish greased with the remaining olive oil. Bake for 30–40 minutes, until cooked.

- In a stockpot, bring stock to a boil. Add the meatballs; cover and simmer for 10 minutes.
- Beat the 2 remaining eggs in a mixing bowl; slowly add lemon juice and some of the hot stock in slow streams as you beat them to achieve a frothy mix.
- Pour egg-lemon mix into the pot with the meatballs. Cover and simmer for another 2–3 minutes and serve immediately.

AUBERGINE MEAT ROLLS

Serves 4–6

- 1 large, round eggplant
- 1 large white onion, finely diced
- 1/2 cup Greek extra-virgin olive oil, divided 2 cloves garlic, minced or pressed
- 1 pound lean ground veal
- 1/2 cup white wine (or Retsina)
- 2 cups strained tomato pulp/juice
- 1 teaspoon ground cumin
- Salt and pepper to taste
- Flour for dredging
- 1 cup shredded or grated Greek Graviera cheese (or mild Gruyère)
- 1/3 cup dried bread crumbs 2 tablespoons finely chopped fresh mint
- 1/3 cup pine nuts 1 egg

Directions

- Preheat the oven to 350°F.

- Wash eggplant thoroughly and remove stalk. Slice thinly along its length; aim for 12 slices. Salt both sides and spread in a flower pattern in a colander. Set aside to drain for 30 minutes. Remember to flip the slices at least once for better drainage.

- In a large frying pan over medium-high heat, sauté onions in 1/4 cup olive oil until soft; stir garlic in for 1 minute. Add meat and mix well; sauté for 8–10 minutes to brown it thoroughly. Set aside while you prepare tomato sauce.

- Add wine, 2 cups tomato juice, cumin, salt, and pepper to a small pot; stir well to mix completely. Bring to a boil and simmer over medium-low heat for 30 minutes, stirring occasionally. Once sauce has completely reduced, remove frying pan from heat and set aside to cool.

- Heat 3 tablespoons olive oil in a large fry pan. Lightly flour both sides of the eggplant slices; fry in batches until softened. Add olive oil to pan as needed, but do it in a thin stream around the entire circumference of the pan so it seeps toward the center. Shake the frying pan back and forth with each batch to keep eggplant slices from sticking to the bottom. Once the eggplant slices have been lightly fried, spread on paper towels in a pan.

- Retrieve the cooled meat mixture. In a large mixing bowl, add cheese (leave aside a few tablespoonfuls of shredded cheese for use as a garnish later), bread crumbs, mint, pine nuts, and egg; mix well to combine with meat. Pick up an eggplant slice; place a heaping spoonful of meat mixture in the middle of one end. Roll up that end to complete a full end-to-end overlapping roll; use a toothpick to pin in place. Be sure not to press the center of the roll too hard, as you do not want the meat to protrude from the open sides.

- Place rolls side by side in close rows in a deep-walled pan greased with olive oil. Spoon tomato sauce on top of rolls in single stripe right along the middle of the rolled slices; sprinkle cheese on top of the tomato sauce stripe.

- Bake for 30 minutes. Let stand to cool for at least 10 minutes before serving. Garnish with a little more shredded cheese while still warm.

PORK WITH LEEKS AND CELERY

Serves 4

- 2 pounds pork shoulder, chopped into cubes
- 1 onion, finely chopped
- 1/2 cup extra-virgin olive oil 1/2 cup white wine 2 cups water
- 2 pounds leeks
- 1 cup finely chopped celery
- 1 cup tomatoes, diced and sieved (fresh or canned)
- 1 teaspoon dried oregano

- Salt and fresh-ground pepper

Directions

- Wash pork well; chop into cubes and set aside to drain.
- In a deep-walled pot, sauté onion in olive oil until slightly soft; add pork and brown thoroughly.
- Add wine to the pot; bring to a boil, then cover and simmer for 15 minutes, stirring regularly. Remove pork; cover to keep warm and set aside.
- Add water to the pan along with the leeks and celery; bring to a boil and simmer for 30 minutes over medium heat.
- Return pork to the pot along with tomatoes, oregano, salt, and pepper; stir well. Bring to a boil and continue to simmer until the sauce is reduced and thickened, approximately 8–10 minutes. Serve immediately.

STIFADO (BRAISED BEEF WITH ONIONS)

Serves 4

- 1⁄2 cup extra-virgin olive oil 2 pounds stewing beef, cubed
- 2 tablespoons tomato paste, diluted in 2 cups of water
- 2 tablespoons wine vinegar (or a sweet dessert wine like Madeira or Mavrodaphne)
- 16 pearl onions, peeled
- 6 cloves garlic, peeled
- 4 spice cloves
- 1 small cinnamon stick

- 1 tablespoon dried oregano
- Salt and fresh-ground pepper

Directions

- Add olive oil to a large pot over medium-high heat; add meat and brown well on all sides by stirring continuously so meat does not stick to the bottom of the pot.
- Add tomato paste, wine vinegar, onions, garlic, cloves, cinnamon, oregano, salt, and pepper; mix well and turn heat to high. Bring to a boil.
- Cover and turn heat down to medium-low; simmer for approximately 1 hour.
- Serve immediately, accompanied by fresh bread for sauce.

BRAISED LAMB SHOULDER

Serves 4

- 1⁄2–2 pounds lamb shoulder
- 1⁄2 cup extra-virgin olive oil
- 1⁄2 cup hot water
- 2 cups tomatoes, diced and sieved (fresh or canned)
- 2 bay leaves
- 4 cloves garlic, peeled and minced
- 1 cinnamon stick
- 1 tablespoon dried thyme
- Salt and pepper to taste

Directions

- Wash meat well and cut into small pieces; include bones.
- Heat olive oil in a pot; brown meat on all sides.

- Add water, tomatoes, bay leaves, garlic, cinnamon, thyme, salt, and pepper; cover and bring to a boil, then turn heat down to medium-low.
- Simmer for 1½ hours, stirring occasionally.

APRICOT-STUFFED PORK TENDERLOIN

Serves 6

- 1½-pound pork tenderloin 1 shallot
- 3 cloves garlic
- 6 apricots
- ½ cup pecans
- 3 fresh sage leaves
- Fresh-cracked black pepper, to taste
- Kosher salt, to taste
- Cooking spray

Directions

- Preheat the oven to 375°F.
- Butterfly the tenderloin by making a lengthwise slice down the middle, making certain not to cut completely through.
- Mince the shallot and garlic. Remove pits and slice apricots. Chop the pecans and sage.
- Lay out the tenderloin. Layer all ingredients over the tenderloin and season with pepper and salt. Carefully roll up the loin and tie securely.
- Spray a rack with cooking spray, then place the tenderloin on the rack and roast for 1–1½ hours. Let cool slightly, then slice.

STEWED SHORT RIBS OF BEEF

Serves 6

- 12 plum tomatoes
- 2 large yellow onions
- 1½ pounds short ribs of beef
- 1 tablespoon ground cumin Fresh-cracked black pepper, to taste
- 1 tablespoon olive oil
- 1 cup dry red wine
- 1 quart Hearty Red Wine Brown Stock

Directions

- Preheat the oven to 325°F.
- Chop the tomatoes. Roughly chop the onions. Season the ribs with cumin and pepper.
- Heat the oil over medium-high heat in a Dutch oven, and sear the ribs on all sides. Add the onions and sauté for 2 minutes, then add the tomatoes and sauté 1 minute more. Add the wine and let reduce by half.
- Add the stock. When stock begins to boil, cover and place in oven for 1– 1½ hours.
- Drain the ribs and vegetables, reserving the stock. Keep the ribs and vegetables warm. Place the stock on the stove over high heat and let the sauce thicken to a gravy-type consistency.

SICILIAN STUFFED STEAK

Serves 6

- 1 pound fresh baby spinach
- 5 eggs, divided

- 1 small yellow onion
- 4 cloves garlic
- 1/2 bunch Italian parsley 1/2 cup olive oil, divided
- 1/2 cup grated pecorino Romano cheese 1/4 pound ground veal Kosher salt, to taste
- Fresh-cracked black pepper
- 2-pound round steak
- 1/2 pound prosciutto, diced
- 1/2 pound provolone or Asiago cheese, diced
- 1 cup dry red wine
- 1 cup veal stock
- 2 teaspoons tomato paste

Directions

- Place the spinach in a saucepan and gently steam over medium heat until tender, about 8–10 minutes. Remove from heat and let cool. Drain and squeeze out as much water as possible.
- Hard-boil 3 of the eggs, peel, and set aside. Finely dice the onion and mince the garlic. Chop the parsley.
- Heat 1/4 cup of the oil over medium heat in a sauté pan; sauté the onion and garlic until golden. Set aside.
- Preheat the oven to 350°F.
- Mix together the Romano cheese, ground veal, parsley, onion, and garlic. Season with salt and pepper. Add the 2 raw eggs and mix again. Spread the mixture evenly over the round steak. Place the slices of hard-boiled eggs in a row on top of the meat and the cheese mixture. Top with diced prosciutto, provolone, and spinach. Roll the meat tightly over stuffing and tie with string to secure it during cooking.
- Brown the meat in the remaining oil until browned all over. Place in an ovenproof pan. In a saucepan, bring the wine, stock, and tomato paste to a boil. Pour this mixture over the meat and roast in the oven for 1 1/2–2 hours, until the internal temperature reaches 165°F. Turn the meat often to baste.
- Remove the meat from the pan and let stand for about 10 minutes before removing the string. Cut into slices and serve with the remaining juices.

SAUSAGE PATTIES

Serves 6
- 2 ounces pork fat
- 2 ounces pancetta
- 1/2 pound ground pork
- 1/2 pound ground veal 1 egg
- 1 tablespoon fresh-cracked black pepper, to taste 1 tablespoon dried sage
- 1/4 teaspoon dried red pepper flakes
- 1 teaspoon ground cumin Kosher salt, to taste
- 1 tablespoon olive oil

Directions

- Finely dice the pork fat and pancetta. Mix together all the ingredients except the oil until thoroughly blended; form into patties.

- Heat the oil over medium heat in a skillet. Brown the patties on each side, covered with a lid to ensure thorough cooking. Drain on a rack lined with paper towels, then serve.

Healthy Beef and Broccoli

Total time: 25 minutes

Prep time: 5 minutes

Cook time: 20 minutes

Ingredients

- 8ml vegetable oil, divided
- 100g flank steak, thinly sliced
- 7.5g corn starch
- 90g broccoli florets
- 60ml water
- 1 green onion, thinly sliced
- 1/2 shallots, finely chopped
- 1 small cloves garlic, minced
- 1g crushed red pepper flakes
- 1g minced fresh ginger
- 5ml honey
- 20 ml soy sauce

Directions

- Add oil to a skillet set over medium heat.
- Stir in beef and cook for about 8 minutes or until browned.
- Remove the beef from the pan and set aside.
- Add green onions, shallots and garlic to the same pan and cook for 1 minute, stirring.
- Stir in broccoli and cook for about 5 minutes.

- Combine cornstarch and water in a mixing bowl until well blended.
- In a separate bowl, combine red pepper flakes, ginger, honey, and soy sauce; stir in the cornstarch mixture until well combined.
- Add sauce to the pan and cook for about 5 minutes or until thick.
- Stir in beef and cook for about 3 minutes.
- Serve over brown rice.

MEDITERRANEAN PIZZA RECIPES

Mediterranean Veggie Pizza

Total time: 27 minutes

Prep time: 15 minutes

Cook time: 12 minutes

Yield: 4 servings

Ingredients

- 1 tbsp. cornmeal
- 1 can refrigerated pizza dough
- 2 tbsp. commercial pesto
- ½ cup mozzarella cheese, shredded
- 1 pack frozen artichoke hearts, thawed, drained and coarsely chopped
- 1 ounce prosciutto, thinly sliced
- 2 tbsp. Parmesan, shredded
- 1 ½ cups Arugula leaves
- 1 ½ tbsp. fresh lemon juice
- Cooking spray

Directions

- Preheat your oven to 500°F.

- Meanwhile, coat a baking sheet with cooking spray and sprinkle with cornmeal.
- Place the dough on the baking sheet by rolling it out.
- Evenly spread the pesto on the dough leaving out close to half an inch from the edge.
- Add the mozzarella over the pesto and now put the baking sheet on the bottom rack of the oven and bake for 5 minutes.
- Add the artichokes onto the pizza plus prosciutto and Parmesan then return the baking sheet to the oven and bake for another 5 – 6 minutes.
- In a small bowl, mix the arugula and the lemon juice and use this to top the pizza.
- You are ready to serve.

Turkish-Style Pizza

Total time: 45 minutes

Prep time: 30 minutes

Cook time: 15 minutes

Yield: 1 14 by 9-inch pizza

Ingredients

- 1 tsp. extra virgin-olive oil, plus 1 tbsp., divided
- Cornmeal, for dusting
- 12 ounces whole-wheat pizza dough
- 1 ½ cups grated Monterey Jack cheese or fontina
- 1 cup diced sweet onion
- 1 ½ cups diced tomatoes
- 2 tbsp. minced seeded jalapeno pepper
- 2 ounces sliced pastrami, diced
- Freshly ground pepper
- ⅓ cup fresh flat-leaf parsley, chopped

Directions

- Position an inverted baking sheet on the lower oven rack and preheat to 500°F.
- Lightly oil a large baking sheet and dust with the cornmeal.
- Lightly flour a clean work surface and roll the dough into 10×15-inch oval.
- Transfer the rolled dough to the baking sheet and fold edges under to form a rim.
- Brush the rim with about 1 teaspoon of extra virgin olive oil.
- Sprinkle the crust with grated cheese, leaving about ½-inch border and top with onion, tomatoes, jalapeno, pastrami, and pepper.
- Drizzle with the remaining extra virgin oil and bake in the preheated oven for about 14 minutes or until the bottom is golden and crisp.
- Serve the pizza warm sprinkled with chopped parsley.

CPSIA information can be obtained
at www.ICGtesting.com
Printed in the USA
BVHW061037220621
610126BV00006B/551